Praise for *Brain Medicine*

In *Brain Medicine,* Rohn outlines the utility of gene editing in combatting anxiety and depression. Using clear illustrations, Rohn explains to a lay readership what's involved in gene therapy, which uses CRISPR (clustered regularly interspaced short palindromic repeats) technology to introduce corrective proteins into broken or problematic gene segments. Readers previously unaware of this incredible new technology will find their imaginations firing when contemplating its potential; they'll likely agree with Rohn that the 21st century could prove to be the Golden Age of medicine. A confident, readable breakdown of the current state of therapeutic gene therapy.

—Kirkus Reviews

Finally, a book that establishes how the nervous system and psychology come together. Want to understand how far the medical field has come in treating anxiety and similar conditions? Start here.

—Noail Isho, MD, neurologist

Dr. Rohn is a medical researcher and professional science communicator who was afflicted by a complex neurological condition and subsequently embarked on a personal search for a cure. There is no better narrator to convey the complexities of the human mind and the intricacies of experimental design in the modern era of drug development.

—Ryan Holzer, Ph.D., founder and director, Rosetta Institute of Biomedical Research

---

Dr. Rohn guides us through the wonders of modern science and the possibilities of personalized gene therapy through sharing his lived experience of anxiety. He does so without shying away from discussing future ethical considerations and the realities of the interactions between modern science, public opinion and public policy. *Brain Medicine* left me motivated to continue to advocate for my patients and excited about the possibilities of modern medicine."

—Ryan Day, MD, primary care internal medicine physician

Brain Medicine represents a thoughtful and rigorously grounded contribution to the neuroscience of anxiety and neuropsychiatric disorders, integrating empirical research with clinically informed insight. This work is a meaningful and impactful resource for scholars, clinicians, and anyone interested in neuroscience-informed approaches to complex neurological disorders.

—Jamison Lee, Ph.D. candidate in
Neuropsychiatry Disorders

In *Brain Medicine*, Dr. Rohn presents gene therapy as a new frontier in the treatment of anxiety. Integrating groundbreaking scientific insight with his own lived experience, he offers a compassionate and authentic vision for the future of neuropsychiatric care.

—Tanner Pollock, MS, CGC

This story of a scientist's quest to develop new treatments for chronic anxiety helps to humanize mental illness and provides personal insight into the process of scientific discovery and the challenges of drug development. In *Brain Medicine*, Dr. Rohn offers a hopeful yet honest assessment of the exciting potential of gene therapy for the treatment of neuropsychiatric disease, even as he addresses the important ethical issues we must consider as these new technologies emerge. Throughout the book, Dr. Rohn describes complex concepts in cellular, molecular, and systems neuroscience using relatable, often comical analogies which are sure to keep readers entertained as they learn about the cutting-edge techniques opening new frontiers in medicine.

—Ben Sachs, Professor of Neuroscience, Villanova University

I had the pleasure of reviewing *Brain Medicine* by Troy Rohn. With 18 years of experience in the mental health field—and living with Generalized Anxiety Disorder myself—I found this book both enlightening and deeply personal. Dr. Rohn skillfully weaves his own story with clear, accessible science, offering a fascinating look at how genetics and neurobiology may shape anxiety and how emerging gene-based therapies could transform treatment. This book brings both insight and hope to anyone seeking a deeper understanding of anxiety and its future care.

—Patrick Fithin, CEO, A Body & Mind

From the world's leading authority on a new class of precision genetic anxiolytic medicines comes the story of how he overcame his personal anxiety issues, going on to pioneer a new solution that could improve the lives of millions of others struggling with anxiety around the globe. *Brain Medicine* is a beacon of hope for anyone who suffers from anxiety or has a family member who does. Anyone living with anxiety now can look forward to a future where there is a solution. We will never stop until we get there. And with brilliant, dedicated scientists like Troy Rohn, we will.

—John L. Mee, founder and president, Cognigenics, Inc.

Brain Medicine is a compelling read that details the use of cutting-edge molecular biology to improve the lives of millions who live with debilitating anxiety. The complicated biochemistry behind CRISPR technology is explained with analogies that even nonscientists will understand.

—Tara Rothwell, PA-C, MS, MPAS

BRAIN MEDICINE

BRAIN MEDICINE

BREAKTHROUGHS IN GENE THERAPY FOR ANXIETY & OTHER NEUROPSYCHIATRIC DISORDERS

TROY ROHN, PhD

Foreword by Dean Radin, PhD

Hatherleigh Press, Ltd.
62545 State Highway 10, Hobart, NY 13788, USA
hatherleighpress.com

BRAIN MEDICINE

Library of Congress Cataloging-in-Publication Data is available.

ISBN: 978-1-961293-66-3

Interior and cover design by Carolyn Kasper

Printed in the United States
The authorized representative in the EU for product safety and compliance is Catarina Astrom, Blästorpsvägen 14, 276 35 Borrby, Sweden. info@hatherleighpress.com

10 9 8 7 6 5 4 3 2 1

Contents

Part III: Breaking Barriers in Brain Health & Gene Therapy

Foreword by Dean Radin, PhD

What motivates a person to become a scientist? For many, it is a deep curiosity about the world, the thrill of solving mysteries, or the desire to make a meaningful impact.

However, for others, the drive to pursue science is deeply personal, born out of their own struggles and the hope to help others overcome similar challenges. Dr. Troy Rohn's journey exemplifies this deeply personal motivation. His battle with chronic anxiety, a condition that can overshadow every moment of life, did not define him—it propelled him toward groundbreaking discoveries that could transform how we understand and treat mental health disorders.

Chronic anxiety is not just a fleeting sense of worry; it is an all-consuming state that affects every aspect of life. For sufferers, the world can feel like a minefield where even the simplest tasks are fraught with potential triggers. Dr. Rohn knows this struggle intimately. His life was shaped by traumatic events, from a difficult childhood to life-threatening experiences as a young adult, leaving him with the lasting imprint of PTSD. The rewiring of his nervous system left him in a state of constant hypervigilance, where stress and fear were ever-present. Yet, instead of being crushed by the weight of this anxiety, Dr. Rohn turned his challenges into motivation for innovation.

Dr. Rohn's path could have led him in many directions, but his resilience and determination set him apart. He refused to let anxiety define his future. Instead, he pursued a career in science, combining his personal experiences with a profound understanding of biology to tackle the root causes of anxiety. This journey was not just about personal healing; it was about finding solutions for countless others who live with similar burdens.

The science of anxiety involves a complex interplay of genetic, environmental, and neurological factors. The brain's network of neurons and neurotransmitters—particularly serotonin, GABA, and others—plays a critical role in regulating mood and anxiety. In anxiety disorders, this delicate balance is disrupted, leading to persistent fear and emotional distress. Dr. Rohn's expertise allowed him to delve into the molecular and genetic underpinnings of these processes, providing new insights into how anxiety manifests and persists.

Traditional treatments for anxiety, such as cognitive-behavioral therapy, meditation, and commonly prescribed medications (such as SSRIs or benzodiazepines), have helped many people. Yet these approaches often fall short. Medications can come with significant side effects and only manage symptoms without addressing the underlying causes. Other methods, like mindfulness or cognitive-behavioral therapy, require substantial time and effort, which can be daunting for individuals already overwhelmed by their condition. Dr. Rohn recognized the need for a different approach, one that could target anxiety at its source.

Dr. Rohn's groundbreaking work in gene therapy represents a monumental shift in how we think about mental health treatment. Leveraging revolutionary gene-editing tools like CRISPR and RNA interference, his research focuses on editing or silencing specific genes involved in anxiety regulation. This approach moves beyond merely treating symptoms; it aims to address the biological roots of anxiety, offering the potential for lasting relief.

In this book, Dr. Rohn discusses the development of two promising therapies he helped develop that reduce anxiety with unprecedented precision and without the many undesirable side effects of traditional drugs.

The results of these therapies in preclinical trials were remarkable. Animal studies have shown both significant reductions in anxiety-related behaviors and astonishingly substantial improvements in memory and cognitive function. These findings suggest that genetic therapies could provide a long-term solution for chronic anxiety, bringing hope to millions of individuals who struggle with this condition. Dr. Rohn's work not only advances the field of mental health treatment but also redefines what is possible.

What makes Dr. Rohn's story so compelling is not just his scientific achievements but the personal journey that brought him to this point. He has lived through the challenges of chronic anxiety and understands its impact on every facet of life. This dual perspective—as both a scientist and a survivor—gives his work a unique depth and authenticity. He does not just approach anxiety as a problem to solve; he approaches it with empathy and a commitment to creating meaningful change.

By sharing candid anecdotes about his own experiences, Dr. Rohn provides a raw and honest account of how it has shaped his life. These stories highlight the resilience required to live with chronic anxiety and speak to those who may feel alone in their struggles. At the same time, the book provides a clear and accessible explanation of the biological science underlying anxiety, making complex concepts understandable to readers without a scientific background.

One of the most exciting aspects of this work is its focus on the future. The potential for genetic therapies to transform mental health treatment is immense, but the road ahead is not without challenges. Dr. Rohn outlines the rigorous process of conducting clinical trials with human patients, the significant costs involved (up to a billion dollars to get a new therapeutic treatment to market), and the regulatory hurdles that must be overcome to gain government approval. He also addresses the ethical considerations of genetic editing, emphasizing the importance of ensuring these innovations are both accessible and equitable.

Dr. Rohn's journey is a testament to the power of perseverance and the transformative potential of science. He has turned his own adversity into a source of inspiration and innovation. His work not only offers hope to those who suffer from anxiety but also serves as a powerful example of how personal struggles can lead to groundbreaking discoveries.

As you read *Brain Medicine*, you will gain a deeper understanding of anxiety, not just as a clinical condition but as a lived experience. You will also learn about the cutting-edge science that holds the promise of changing how we approach mental health treatment. Most importantly, you will see how one person's determination and vision can pave the way for a brighter future for millions of people.

—Dean Radin, PhD

Preface

One of the time-honored traditions of being a professor is the sabbatical. Most major universities offer some form of a sabbatical, such as a paid leave of absence to focus on scholarly activity. At my home institution, one can apply every seven years.

In my case, I had never taken a sabbatical in the 25 years I had taught for a state university. Unfortunately, these opportunities do not roll over, and 2024 felt like the right time to take advantage of this quirky professional opportunity. My responsibilities included teaching a full range of courses, from non-major Biology 100 to graduate-level molecular neuroscience. I still have a dedicated research program involving Alzheimer's disease. Together with teaching, these experiences have honed my writing skills to clearly communicate complex scientific concepts, and I have authored 80 peer-reviewed articles.

My goal during this sabbatical was to use my time free from my standard university duties to focus on our biotech start-up company, Cognigenics, which I helped build beginning in 2019. At Cognigenics, our focus is on applying gene therapy approaches to treat neurological disorders, including anxiety and memory impairments.

At the time, I anticipated our company swimming in capital ($10 million) based on our robust preclinical results. However, that has yet to be the case. As the saying goes in the movie *Field of Dreams*, I believed that "If you build it, they will come." The cold reality, though, is that building a strong science base and thinking financial resources will automatically flow in is difficult, especially in the volatile venture capital world.

These challenges have made me more determined to share my story. Being an individual who has gone through the process of experiencing the ecstasy and the agony of innovation while struggling with anxiety as a real-life issue, I believe I offer a unique point of view. This is not just a book about science and how we can change the world with it. It is about the intersection of personal experience, persistence, and the promise of groundbreaking therapies. As such, it is a story that only I can tell.

In truth, writing a book was intended as a way to narrate a cathartic experience of my demons with anxiety, as well as my determination to find better treatments for this disabling disorder. As the title suggests, this book is not only about the science behind gene therapy and its potential application in treating neurological disorders such as anxiety, but also about the personal experiences that have inspired me to find better treatments. As a neuroscientist, I recognize that most human behaviors result from a combination of genetic and environmental factors, and my experiences are no exception.

I hope my story and a greater understanding of the mechanics of gene therapy will inspire and enlighten readers. I invite you to share in the excitement of how gene therapy is set to become the landmark medical breakthrough of the twenty-first century, offering solutions and ushering in what I believe will be the Golden Age of Medicine.

—Troy Rohn, PhD

Part I

Anatomy of Anxiety: From Personal Struggles to Molecular Pathways

1

Me, Worry?

My Anxiety Journey

ANXIETY DISORDERS TEND to run in families because of genetic influences. This means that if someone in the family has been diagnosed with anxiety, depression, or other mental health problems, it is more likely that another family member will also experience anxiety. Studies reveal that the genetic component for anxiety disorders falls between 30 and 50 percent, indicating that a substantial portion of the risk is passed down through our genes.

In addition, early childhood experiences like trauma, abuse, or neglect have been shown to significantly increase the chances of developing anxiety disorders. Stressful events within the family dynamic can even disturb the normal growth of emotional control, making these children more vulnerable to anxiety problems later in life.

As someone who experiences anxiety, I have tried to look back on my childhood and early adulthood in order to reflect on and understand better why I react the way I do. This chapter presents my story.

Living around alcoholism and addiction can impact *any* facet of life. If you are concerned that reading about this behavior might be triggering, *please stop here* and continue your reading in Chapter 2. Shorter vignettes are also included at the beginning of each chapter.

FAMILY DYNAMICS

Growing up, my family dynamics were less like *Leave It to Beaver* and more like a Netflix true-crime drama in the making. My mom and all of those in her orbit struggled with addiction, and I was severely traumatized by their erratic behavior. I remember on several occasions helping my mom barricade our front door against my mother's second husband's entry, following his night of heavy drinking at the local Moose Lodge. It was not uncommon for the local sheriff to show up at our home during such disputes. When I was ten years old, my grandmother took me aside to tell me that Mom's husband was not my biological father and that my biological father died in an automobile accident.

In addition to this distress, we were nearly destitute. Following her second divorce, my mom spent a few years taking care of three children on a meager salary, and I had numerous meetings with our school principal regarding my "anger issues." By the time my mom's third husband came into the picture, well, let's just say that her decision to remarry did not go over well.

My sisters and I were often left alone for days in an isolated rural area. Spending the night alone was terrifying for me, as was the threat of punishment after my mother returned. (During my high school years, my mom finally became sober; however, by that time, the damage was done.)

During my doctoral studies at the University of Washington, I hit a nadir. Fortunately, through counseling, I realized that although my mother provided shelter and nourishment, she did little else to support me as a child. Self-blame for my lack of love towards her should not have been on my shoulders. That revelation was mind-blowing, and I immediately felt a weight lifted.

DIAGNOSIS

I gained another vital insight from counseling: It is virtually impossible to experience child abuse and neglect without mental harm. While anxiety initially lurked beneath the surface, manifesting subtly, it was not disruptive enough to affect my daily life. However, in retrospect, it was clear that the effect was quite significant, especially in the case of my interpersonal relationships, or rather in my lack thereof.

Let me provide a couple of concrete examples. I despise being in crowds of unknown people (at a concert, for example). For me, going to a music concert represents sheer terror and anxiety. But here's the thing: once I participated in a concert, I realized it was not *that bad*, and I even enjoyed the event.

I used to attend at least one professional conference per year. But as my anxiety became worse, I found myself attending these conferences but then literally locking myself in my hotel room and avoiding interactions with my peers at all costs. (On the lighter side, I did perfect my hotel room's coffee maker operation and became intimately familiar with every pay-per-view option available!)

Everything came to a head during and after the COVID pandemic. At that time, the prevalence of depression and anxiety increased by *three to four times* among U.S. adults (Cai et al., 2021; Twenge et al., 2021). I began to suffer from severe anxiety and sought additional counseling as recommended by my family doctor.

Through several counseling sessions, I gained a deeper understanding of the anxiety I had been experiencing.

THREE-PART TREATMENT: COGNITIVE-BEHAVIORAL THERAPY, SERVICE ANIMALS & MEDICATION

Among other things, I learned about "situational anxiety." Per the *Diagnostic and Statistical Manual of Mental Disorders (5th ed.)* (DSM-5), situational anxiety pertains to feelings of anxiety that arise in response to circumstances or occurrences rather than being classified as a separately diagnosable condition. Instead, it is typically viewed as a symptom associated with other anxiety disorders, like social anxiety disorder or generalized anxiety disorder.

Anxiety, in situations, often arises due to stress triggers such as:

- Career interviews
- Traveling by airplane
- Examinations
- Encountering individuals

The level of anxiety experienced in the circumstances can differ significantly in strength—from unease to intense panic episodes—based on an individual's sensitivity and the specific situation at hand.

My first step in treatment involved a type of therapy called **Cognitive Behavioral Therapy (CBT).** This is a common approach used to help people understand and change the patterns of thinking or behavior that contribute to their anxiety. At first, the name CBT sounded intimidating, but it's really just a structured way to help people recognize and change negative thought patterns that contribute to anxiety. Instead of letting worries spiral out of control, CBT helps replace unhelpful thoughts with more constructive ones.

One of the best things about CBT is that it doesn't rely on medication. It's a hands-on, problem-solving approach that teaches real strategies to handle stressful situations. I found it especially useful because it gave me practical tools I could use whenever anxiety crept up.

HOW DOES CBT WORK?

One of the most effective CBT techniques is visualization, which is like mentally rehearsing a situation before it happens. By imagining a stressful scenario in a controlled way, you can train your brain to handle it more calmly in real life. It's a little like preparing for a big speech—practicing in your head makes it easier when the moment comes.

For instance, one of my biggest anxiety triggers was being in large crowds. Concerts, conferences, airports—whatever it was, they all made me nervous. However, I didn't want to miss out on experiences just because of my anxiety. So, I used CBT to practice mental exposure therapy, which involves picturing myself in the situation beforehand so that it wouldn't feel so overwhelming when it actually happened.

A great test for this was seeing Dave Matthews at the Gorge—one of my favorite bands in one of the most beautiful concert venues in the world!

Here's how I used CBT to prepare:

- I imagined the entire process step by step—arriving at the venue, walking through the crowds, finding my seat, and feeling the excitement in the air.
- I envisioned myself managing each moment with calm, reminding myself that the experience was meant to be enjoyed, not feared.
- I thought through possible challenges (like bumping into a sea of strangers) and visualized myself managing them with ease.

By the time I actually went to the concert, I felt ready. My anxiety didn't disappear completely, but it was manageable. Instead of dreading the experience, I actually enjoyed it!

Of course, I had an important secret weapon—my wife, Lisa, who supported me through it all. Having her there made a huge difference, but so did the preparation.

Instead of avoiding concerts altogether, CBT gave me the confidence to face them head-on.

In addition to CBT, I now have a service dog, Bailey, trained in **deep pressure therapy (DPT).** I had known from my teachings in neuroscience that service dogs can be indispensable for people suffering from anxiety disorders such as PTSD. Applying pressure to their owner's bodies—often by leaning against them—can induce a sense of calmness and stability similar to the soothing effects of weighted blankets.

In research conducted in 2018 on the advantages of service dogs, war veterans shared their experiences about how the gentle nudges from their service dogs helped them during flashback moments. These interactions helped in managing their PTSD by breaking the cycle and bringing them back to reality. Service dogs also remind veterans to stay focused on the moment (Yarborough et al., 2018).

In addition, according to a study by Lass-Hennemann and colleagues, having a service dog can significantly reduce stress levels in challenging situations (Lass-Hennemann et al., 2014). This discovery is backed by other research indicating that service dogs can help lower physical and mental stress levels, ultimately improving overall health and happiness.

Finally, a more recent study highlighted the effectiveness of this kind of therapy, whereby the authors convincingly linked the pairing of service dogs with lowered PTSD severity, the odds of diagnosis, and other adverse mental health problems in military veterans (Leighton et al., 2024).

The third leg of the treatment stool is medication. Doctors prescribe two major types of anti-anxiety medications: benzodiazepines and selective serotonin reuptake inhibitors (SSRIs). The members of the **benzodiazepine** group include Valium, Xanax, and Ativan, among others. These drugs have been around for a while, making them the standard for anxiety treatment (despite the many controversies that have surrounded them).

Here is how benzodiazepines work: Imagine your brain is hosting a party, and some guests (neurons) are overacting, dancing, yelling, and spilling their drinks.

Benzodiazepines calm the party down by boosting the effects of GABA, a neurotransmitter. Much like the responsible friend, GABA says, "Okay, everybody chill," telling the neurons to relax and making benzodiazepines highly effective at reducing anxiety.

However, just like that friend of yours, benzodiazepines can be problematic. Used for extended periods or in large quantities, it can lead to sedation, confusion, and even withdrawal issues (Olfson et al., 2015). Due to these risks, benzodiazepines are used for a short period of perhaps a few weeks (Baldwin et al., 2013).

This is where **SSRIs** come in. SSRIs are used for the long term because they take their time to start working and have fewer side effects. They affect serotonin levels, a chemical messenger in the brain that helps control mood. In the case of Zoloft, for instance, the doctor will often begin with a low dose (25-50 mg per day) and gradually adjust based on how well it works.

However, as with most medications, there are some issues with SSRIs. They require a daily commitment (no skipping pills!), and they come with a grab bag of side effects. And importantly, they do not work for everyone. Some people—about 30–40 percent—might not see any improvement at all (Jakubovski et al., 2019; Strawn et al., 2015;

Suresh et al., 2020). For those folks, it may be like throwing coins into a well, hoping for something to happen.

Instead of doubling down on meds that only work for some, why not explore new, twenty-first-century possibilities—like gene therapy? Ultimately, this is not just about anxiety; it is about tackling a whole host of neuropsychiatric disorders, from depression to ADHD. Before I get ahead of myself, let's stick with anxiety for now. The science gets even more interesting from here.

2

The Serotonin Solution

Targeting the 5-HT2A Receptor to Rewire Anxiety

ADDICTION CREATES MANY victims. One way it does this is by distorting or denying facts, events, and reality in general.

A recently-discovered box containing dozens of letters from my biological father reveals a broken man who had been manipulated and deceived. The letters included an encounter with a man years after my parents' divorce, with whom my mother had had an affair:

I do not know what happens in [her] mind; her motives are usually black... There are a host of victims in this entire mess, but ... I believe he is too gullible, naive, and weak to ward off the gross manipulation...

My mother (as I gleaned from these letters) also would not allow our father to visit us unless he paid child support and would drive a wedge between him and his children by saying he did not care about us.

My father was not without his problems (financial instability, depression and anxiety, and bouts of alcohol abuse and gambling). Yet, his letters show a very articulate, sensitive person who wanted to have a relationship with his two children. Unfortunately, he never got that chance. On July 16, 1971, he was killed in an automobile accident at the age of 31. I was only four years old.

My mother wrote another disturbing letter to my father. The story goes that I jumped off of the couch, landed awkwardly on the coffee table, and proceeded to break my hip. I was in a body cast for an extended period.

Following the "accident," it took weeks before my mom took me to the hospital, part of a pattern of neglect throughout my infancy, undoubtedly contributing to later PTSD.

BRAIN CIRCUIT THEORY

The letters from my dad were not only parts of a sad story; they became a way for me to understand the origins of my own anxiety: the unhealed trauma, unkindness, and loss.

What I experienced in my childhood influenced the development of my brain, wiring me for hypervigilance and emotional distress.

Based in part on these experiences, I postulate that there exists what I will call a "Hyperactive Distressive Connectome": a network of neural pathways controlling the storage of dysfunctional memories, the processing of negative experiences, and the generation of maladaptive responses. This hypothesis is illustrated in the following wheel diagram (Figure 2.1), which shows this connectome's four major hubs: the amygdala, hippocampus, insular cortex (or insula), and thalamus.

Figure 2.1: The "Hyperactive Distressive Connectome" Hypothesis

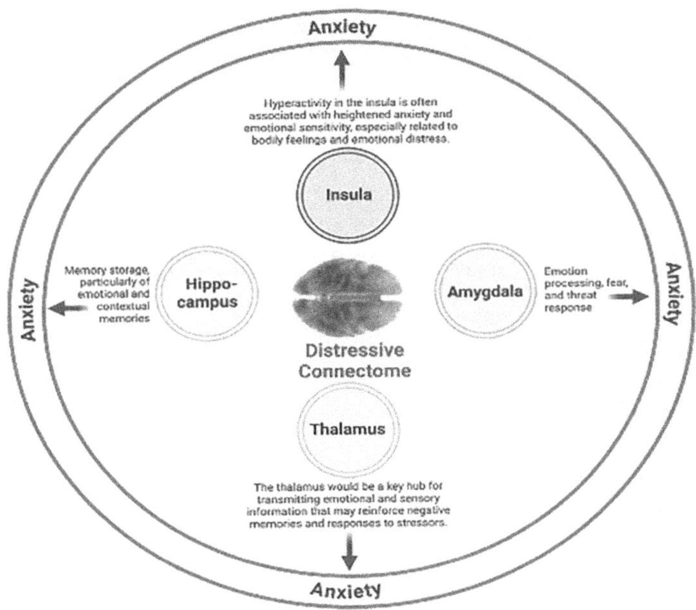

Note: As illustrated, this Connectome involves key brain hubs, including the **insula**, **hippocampus**, **amygdala**, *and* **thalamus**. *When hyperactivity is present in this network, it can perpetuate a cycle of emotional distress, leading to chronic anxiety.*

The **insula** (or insular cortex) is central for coordinating internal body states and emotional experiences. Chronic anxiety can arise when the insula is hyperactive, causing individuals to be overly sensitive to signs such as heartbeat or tense muscles. This increased sensitivity can worsen feelings of anxiety, creating a cycle where anxiety intensifies feelings that, in turn, increase anxiety levels further.

The **hippocampus** is involved in memory formation, affecting emotional and specific environmental cues. If the hippocampus becomes overactive or if memories are constantly retrieved in response to anxiety-provoking situations, it may reinforce the connection between particular stimuli and emotional distress. This could lead to a situation where anxiety is triggered more easily and frequently, further maintaining the chronic nature of the disorder.

The **amygdala** plays a crucial role in emotion processing, especially in the context of fear and threat responses. Hyperactivity in the amygdala is often associated with exaggerated responses to perceived threats. Therefore, individuals with anxiety disorders might experience a response in the amygdala towards harmless stimuli, which can result in prolonged feelings of fear. The constant firing of the amygdala in response to perceived threats can drive ongoing anxiety.

The **thalamus** serves as a hub for relaying input to brain regions. It may intensify sensory signals that feed into the Hyperactive Distressive Connectome if it becomes overly sensitive or hyperactive. Based on this role, hyperactivity of the thalamus can sustain feelings of anxiety over time by processing inputs such as loud noises or excessively crowded environments.

According to my hypothesis, anxiety feeds off the heightened emotional and sensory inputs provided by this network. Each hub then contributes to a vicious cycle where emotional responses (fear, anxiety) and bodily reactions (like increased heart rate or sweating) mutually reinforce each other, leading to chronic anxiety symptoms.

Think of the Hyperactive Distressive Connectome as a group chat you cannot leave. The amygdala is the friend who panics over everything, the hippocampus keeps bringing up old arguments. The insula constantly complains about how bad they feel, and the thalamus spams you with every notification imaginable. Together, they keep your brain in a perpetual state of "Do Not Disturb."

Understanding the hyperactivity of what I have termed the Distressive Connectome opens the door to targeted therapies, including gene therapy. This theory also provides a rationale for focusing on downregulating the excitatory serotonin 5-hydroxytryptamine 2A (5-HT2A) receptor as a potential solution for chronic anxiety and memory impairments.

THE ROLE OF NEUROTRANSMITTERS IN ANXIETY

The human brain is incredibly complex when expressing emotions and is involved in every aspect of emotional processing. Moods are more than feelings; they are the product of an interaction among neural pathways and chemical messengers known as neurotransmitters. These neurotransmitters significantly impact euphoria, sadness, anxiety, irritability, and apathy.

Some key neurotransmitters that play a role in shaping mood include:

- Serotonin
- Dopamine
- Norepinephrine
- GABA

Each has a function in influencing our emotional state. Serotonin is commonly linked with feelings of joy and good spirits. Meanwhile, GABA, in its role, alleviates anxiety and stressors. When these neurotransmitters are out of balance, they can result in different moods, such as joyfulness or sadness, as well as anger or anxiousness.

Studies have shown that serotonin not only affects mood but also has connections to specific anxiety disorders and influences our reactions to situations as well. When the levels of serotonin in the brain go awry, it can result in heightened stress and anxiety levels.

We can think of GABA as a neurotransmitter that helps calm the brain by slowing down neuron activity, bringing about a sense of calmness. This illustrates the importance of GABA in alleviating symptoms associated with anxiety, like muscle tension and restlessness. Conversely, serotonin plays a role in adjusting the thinking aspects of anxiety, like constant worry and fixation, while also regulating emotional reactions to stress.

THE SEROTONIN & GABA BALANCE

Serotonin is recognized for its stimulating effects on neurons compared to the inhibitory nature of the GABA receptor, as shown in Figure 2.2. When serotonin levels rise during moments like being alert or experiencing stress and emotions, it stimulates the activity of neurons, referred to as neuronal spiking activity. In contrast, the role of GABA is essential in toning down this stimulation to maintain a balanced network.

Figure 2.2: Simulated Neuronal Spiking Activity in the Presence of GABA & Serotonin

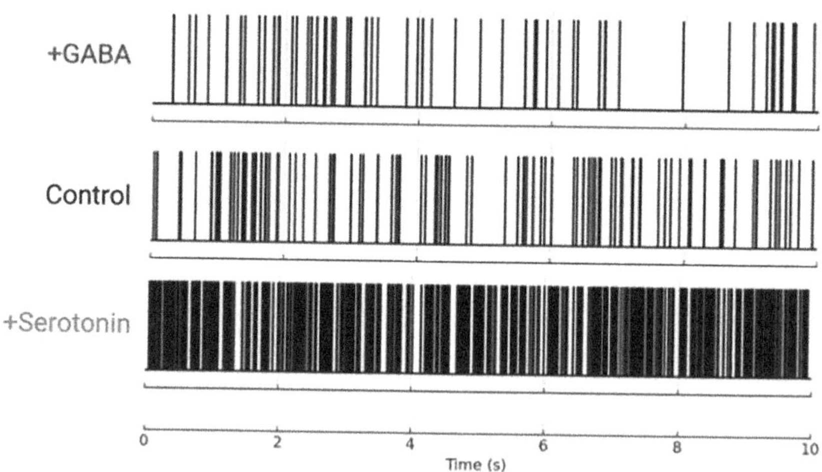

Note: These data do not represent actual data and are for illustration purposes only. The top panel shows neuronal spiking activity with the application of GABA, which acts as an inhibitory neurotransmitter, reducing the frequency of action potentials, the main form of electrical signals used to communicate within the nervous system. The middle panel represents control conditions, demonstrating typical neuronal spiking. The bottom panel shows the effect of serotonin application, which is known to have excitatory effects and lead to an increased frequency of action potentials. This contrast between GABA's inhibitory and serotonin's excitatory actions highlights these neurotransmitters' different modulatory roles in regulating neuronal activity.

THE 5-HT2A RECEPTOR & ANXIETY

The ability of serotonin to act as a mood modulator relies on the specific interaction with membrane-bound protein receptors. This is an essential concept in pharmacology: all biological effects of neurotransmitters are mediated by the interaction between a neurotransmitter and its **receptor**. The two go hand in hand, much like "frick and frack," "ping pong," and "hip hop." When it comes to the impact of serotonin, the key lies not only in the quantity of serotonin released but in the specific subtype of receptor it binds to. What exactly is a receptor?

A receptor protein is akin to a keyhole found on the cell's exterior plasma membrane, and molecules such as serotonin act as the corresponding keys. When the correct key (serotonin) aligns with the lock (receptor), a message is transmitted within the cell to trigger a response. This response may vary from increasing activity, prompting neuron firing, or even causing a slowdown based on the receptor. Due to the properties of the plasma membrane, serotonin cannot cross because of its charged, polar nature.

In the twentieth century, scientists coined the term receptor while investigating the mechanisms of cell interactions with substances. (The word originates from the Latin word "*recipere*," which translates to "to receive" or "to take in.") They observed that cells possess distinct locations, now known as "receptors," where particular molecules, such as hormones or neurotransmitters, bind to initiate a reaction. In this way, receptors act as "receivers" that detect signals. Similar to how a radio picks up frequencies, a receptor reacts solely to specific molecules, with the biological response changing based on which receptor the molecule binds to.

Serotonin receptors act as the "receiving stations," detecting serotonin and facilitating its impact on the brain and body (Figure 2.3).

Figure 2.3: The Serotonin Synapse

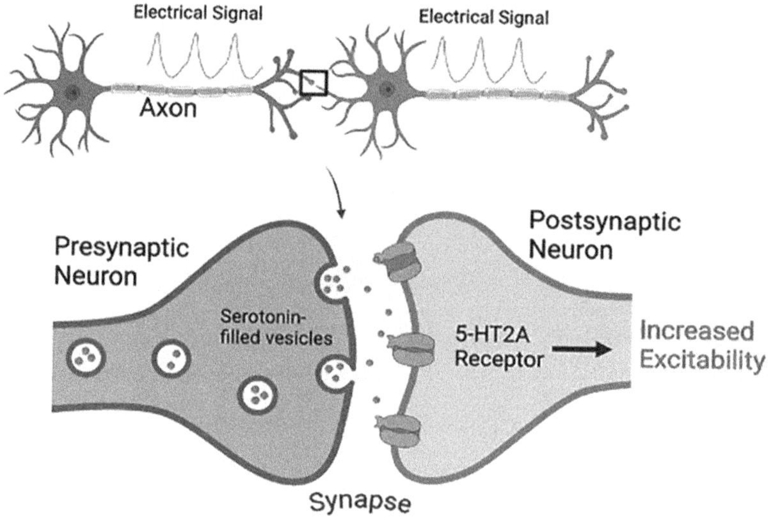

Note: The synapse is a narrow gap between the presynaptic and postsynaptic terminals of adjacent neurons at a synapse. It serves as a physical barrier for transmitting electrical signals between neurons. Neurotransmitters are chemicals that bridge that gap and allow the electrical signal to be converted into a chemical signal. In this case, serotonin is released by the presynaptic neuron

into the synapse, diffusing across the gap to bind with, in this example, 5-HT2A receptors on the postsynaptic neuron, thereby facilitating the transfer of information between neurons. The result is an increased excitability (that is, firing rate) of the postsynaptic neuron.

THE GENE THAT IMPACTS ANXIETY

Notably, there are 15 different types of serotonin receptors commonly referred to as 5-HT receptor subtypes (Berger et al., 2009), representing one of the largest receptor families in the human brain! The terminology 5-HT comes from the structure of serotonin: 5-hydroxytryptophan. (The amino acid tryptophan is the immediate precursor to 5-HT-it explains why people often associate eating foods rich in tryptophan, like turkey, with feeling sleepy or relaxed.)

All 15 subtypes of receptors have different roles in the body and brain. The power of gene therapy is the ability to home in on just one of these: **5-HT2A.**

Out of the 15 kinds of 5-HT receptors in the nervous system, the 5-HT receptor known as 5-HT2A stands out notably due to its strong connection with feelings of anxiety. The 5-HT2A receptor and I have one thing in common: we both get overstimulated under pressure, but only one of us has a therapeutic target on its back.

Also, as you'll read in later chapters, the **gene expression** rule is:

DNA>mRNA>protein

In this case, the flow of genetic information would be:

***HTR2A* gene>5-HTR2A receptor mRNA>**
5-HTR2A protein receptor

A note for readers: By convention, genes are always spelled out in all caps and italicized to differentiate between the RNA messenger and the actual protein.

Anxiety-related disorders, such as generalized anxiety disorder (GAD), panic disorder, post-traumatic stress disorder (PTSD), and social anxiety disorder (SAD), have all been linked to disruptions in communication processes involving the 5-HT2A receptor. For example, research has indicated that when the 5-HT2A receptor is activated in mice experiencing PTSD-related symptoms, it leads to an *increase* in behaviors associated with heightened anxiety (Xiang et al., 2017).

Studies have indicated that receptors such as 5-HT2A also contribute to behaviors related to anxiety and aggression, which suggests that alterations in the functioning of the 5-HT2A receptor may be connected to anxiety issues. One such study showed that using **anti-sense oligonucleotides (AONs)** to target the 5-HT2A receptor decreased rat anxiety levels. This finding supports the receptors' involvement in regulating anxiety levels (Cohen, 2005).

Exploring the impact of manipulating the 5-HT2A receptor pharmacologically has also shown promise as an approach to treating anxiety disorders. One example is the utilization of antipsychotics that typically function as antagonists at the receptor (that is, they inhibit the receptors' ability to link to proteins). It has also been proposed that these drugs help alleviate anxiety symptoms by regulating serotonergic signaling (Erberk-Ozen, 2008).

In a seminal genetic study, scientists disabled the *HTR2A* gene, which encodes the 5-HT2A receptor, and observed that those mice with disabled *HTR2A* genes showed reduced anxiety-related behaviors compared to regular mice (Weisstaub et al., 2006). In other words, when the activity of this receptor was lowered, the mice displayed fewer signs of anxiety in different scenarios, such as exploring open areas or engaging with unfamiliar surroundings.

THE ACTIVITY OF THE 5-HT2A RECEPTOR

Different hypotheses exist for how the overactivation of the 5-HT2A receptor could lead to a heightened anxious state. I'll focus on two.

First Hypothesis

The first hypothesis is that the dysregulation of excitatory and inhibitory networks in the cortex leads to anxiety. Remember, when serotonin binds to the 5-HT2A receptor, it causes the excitation of the corresponding neurons. The imbalance of this process can then cause an increase in activity in regions like the **amygdala**, which (as we know) is closely linked to our fear response to anxiety. This extreme overactivation of the 5-HT2A receptor can amplify how the amygdala reacts to fear and stress, leading to heightened levels of anxiety. The amygdala's primary function is to assist in handling strong negative emotions, like fear, and other instincts related to survival situations. It plays a role in identifying threats and initiating the body's response to fight or flee when faced with danger. Thus, unlike anxious individuals, people with a low-performing amygdala tend to *ignore* fear and dangerous situations.

An extreme example is Alex Honnold, often considered the World's greatest solo climber. He climbed El Capitan in Yosemite National Park without any ropes or protection, and some sports enthusiasts claim this is the most remarkable sporting feat ever. Interestingly, a study comparing his amygdala to rock climbers of a similar age showed it to be inert and non-responsive to fear-inducing images, which may explain his extreme risk-taking behavior (Mackinnon, 2016).

Second Hypothesis

A second hypothesis involves serotonin and the 5-HT2A receptor in the **prefrontal cortex**. The prefrontal cortex serves like a conductor in an orchestra. If all other areas of the brain are instruments in the orchestra but are not in sync, the result is a disaster. The prefrontal cortex helps harmonize the entire brain so that beautiful music can be heard.

In this manner, the prefrontal cortex plays a crucial function in our thinking, decision-making, and planning, and it smoothens our emotional highs and lows. Serotonin and the 5-HT2A receptor work together in the prefrontal cortex to make sure these actions are carried out in a controlled manner. Therefore, overactivation of this receptor can disrupt the prefrontal cortex and its control of emotional regulation, producing heightened anxiety.

PHARMACOLOGIC MECHANISMS

Studies in pharmacology support the association of the 5-HT2A receptor with anxiety. A variety of substances that impact this receptor display both anxiety-reducing and anxiety-inducing effects based on the circumstances and brain area involved. Let us take the case of a 5-HT2A antagonist.

What is a drug antagonist, and how does it work? Think of the receptors in your brain (such as the 5-HT2A receptor) as parking spaces where natural neurotransmitters (like serotonin) are cars meant to park to carry out their functions effectively. When a drug antagonist arrives at the scene, it is akin to another car occupying that designated spot. The car does not perform the function intended, as it is blocked from parking, resulting in a halt to the process. Similarly, the antagonist drug hinders the receptor's operation by taking up its designated space.

Antagonists of the 5-HT2A receptor have demonstrated anxiety-reducing properties. Drugs like mirtazapine and ketanserin, for example, have been shown to alleviate anxiety symptoms in patients. Blocking the 5-HT2A receptors then helps to decrease the neuronal excitability in the cortex and moderates activity in the brain's amygdala and prefrontal cortex regions, resulting in a calming effect.

A second example of pharmacological evidence involves **selective serotonin reuptake inhibitors (SSRIs).** These are some of the most widely used medications for not just anxiety-related disorders but also depression. This class of drugs includes Prozac, the first FDA-approved SSRI (in 1987), Zoloft, Lexapro, Celexa, and Paxil. Currently, 125 million SSRI prescriptions are distributed in the US each year, attesting to their effectiveness.

As their name suggests, SSRIs selectively block the **reuptake transporter** for serotonin. How does this work? When serotonin is released, it is usually recaptured by the sending neuron using this "vacuum cleaner." Recapturing serotonin quickly terminates the receiving response, allowing the sending neuron to reuse the serotonin.

Blocking this reuptake system will, therefore, result in an immediate increase in the available level of serotonin in the synapse (Figure 2.4).

Figure 2.4: Selective Serotonin Reuptake Inhibitor (SSRI) Action

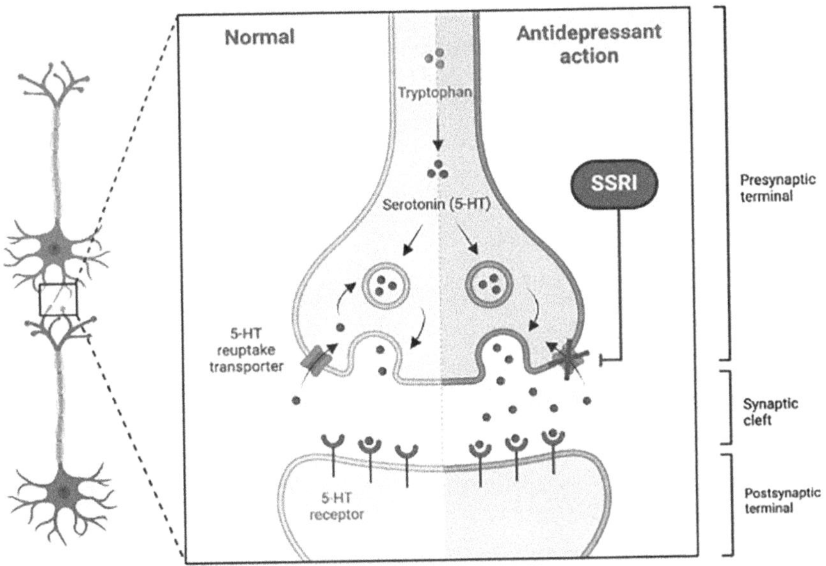

Note: This diagram illustrates the normal function of serotonin (5-HT) in the synaptic cleft and the effect of SSRIs on serotonin reuptake. In a typical synapse, serotonin is released from the presynaptic terminal and binds to 5-HT receptors on the postsynaptic neuron. Usually, serotonin is reabsorbed by the presynaptic neuron via 5-HT reuptake transporters, thus limiting its availability in the synaptic cleft. SSRIs inhibit the 5-HT reuptake transporters, preventing serotonin from being reabsorbed, which increases its concentration in the synaptic cleft and enhances its binding to postsynaptic receptors, resulting in an antidepressant effect.

IMPACT OF MEDICINES ON SYMPTOMS OF ANXIETY

How do SSRIs improve symptoms of anxiety and depression? When I teach this complex topic to my students, it's often not easy for them to grasp. It is an oversimplification to suggest that SSRIs make you feel better by increasing the number of serotonin molecules in the synapse, which they do. The problem: It is not uncommon for patients to notice no improvement in their symptoms until between three and ten weeks after beginning medication. This is true even though, *within just 30 minutes of administration*, an SSRI would be increasing the level of serotonin within the synapse.

To reconcile this problem, one must consider the receptors on the receiving end of the neuron. Over time, excessive serotonin levels in the brain prompt a process where specific receptors, such as 5-HT2A, are decreased to maintain equilibrium. This process, known as **down-regulation**, can reduce the total number of 5-HT2A receptors in the brain over time. Down-regulated neurons then alter how serotonin impacts brain function, potentially alleviating anxiety or enhancing mood regulation. For an analogy, imagine your brain is like a busy office with many workers. The serotonin (5-HT) in this analogy is like a manager who walks around the office, giving instructions (signals) to the workers (neurons) to keep things running smoothly.

Now, let's say there's an event where the manager (serotonin) starts giving instructions constantly. At first, the workers (neurons) respond actively, but after a while, they get overwhelmed because the manager is always around, giving too many instructions.

To deal with this constant overload, the workers (neurons) start removing or ignoring some of the manager's (serotonin's) instructions. This is like the workers (neurons) downregulating their response, meaning they "turn down" or reduce their sensitivity to the manager's message. In the brain, this is what happens when the 5-HT2A receptor is downregulated—it becomes less responsive to serotonin over time, especially if there is a lot of serotonin signaling.

So, downregulation is like the workers in the office saying, "We can't keep up with the constant instructions, so we'll just stop listening as much to avoid being overwhelmed."

Herein lies the problem: SSRIs are not selective and boost the serotonin levels at *all* synapses. Therefore, SSRIs can lead to receptor downregulation in any or all 15 serotonin receptor subtypes. In other words, with an SSRI, we cannot pick and choose which serotonin receptor to downregulate. (This also contributes to the side effect profile for this class of drugs, including nausea, diarrhea, indigestion, agitation, irregular heartbeat, sexual ideation, and hallucinations.)

TARGETING THE 5-HT2A RECEPTOR VS. USING CONVENTIONAL MEDICATION

To appreciate the value of targeting the 5-HT2A receptor for anxiety, one can compare our **gene therapy** approach with other conventional methods. The analogy of a construction worker repairing a damaged wall is illustrative. Different materials and tools yield varying results in fixing the wall; some provide temporary fixes, and others offer a more long-term solution. Treating anxiety operates similarly. Various approaches to treating anxiety, such as medication or gene therapy, function uniquely to address the underlying issues. So, the type of treatment chosen can significantly influence the result.

Conventional treatments like SSRIs are frequently the first tools used to address anxiety. These medications function by enhancing levels of serotonin in the brain to enhance mood and alleviate anxiety symptoms.

Nonetheless, this approach is similar to fortifying a wall without first precisely addressing the vulnerable spots in the wall. While it may assist, SSRIs fail to address the specific cause of anxiety. Additionally, it typically takes several weeks or even months to exhibit noticeable improvements. Finally, SSRI medications do not work for everyone and can cause issues, such as tiredness or weight gain, in some individuals.

Alternatively, targeting the 5-HT2A receptor through gene therapy takes a precise route. Gene therapy is a precise way to target the 5-HT2A receptor to the root cause of anxiety without disrupting the entire neural network. Instead of rewiring the entire system, this approach is akin to fixing one faulty circuit in a large electrical grid. Gene therapy can more effectively reduce anxiety with fewer side effects by selectively suppressing the gene that codes for the excessive 5-HT2A receptor.

The following table lays out treatment with medication compared to gene therapy:

Table 2.1: How Traditional Approaches Stack Up to Gene Therapy Targeting the 5-HT2A Receptor

TREATMENT TYPE	EFFECTIVENESS	SPEED OF ACTION	SIDE EFFECTS	PRECISION
SSRIs (e.g. Zoloft)	Moderate for many, with 40 percent of patients classified as treatment-resistant	Slow (weeks to months)	Fatigue, weight gain, sexual dysfunction, others	Low (broad serotonin increase); no reported benefits to memory
Benzodiazepines (e.g. Xanax)	Quick but short-term	Fast (hours)	Marked sedation, high risk of dependency	Moderate (calms overall anxiety); can impair memory
Gene Therapy (5-HT2A Receptor)	High, may also improve memory	Fast (potentially)	Fewer (targeted approach)	High (targets specific receptor); decreases anxiety and improves memory

According to this table, focusing gene therapy on the 5-HT2A receptor affords a notable benefit compared to conventional therapies.

Even though SSRIs might work for some individuals, they can:

- Take a while to show results.
- Lead to various side effects.
- Have a widespread impact on the brain.

Although another class of drugs, benzodiazepines, acts fast, they are not a solution and carry the potential for dependence (Fluyau et al., 2018).

On the other hand, gene therapy offers a more targeted and enduring approach with fewer adverse reactions by focusing on the specific region of the brain most involved in anxiety: the 5-HT2A receptor. The precision of this method is what gives gene therapy its potential promise as a new tool to address anxiety symptoms. Although this method is still in the preclinical stages of development, the possibilities are immense. We can imagine a future where anxiety is not just controlled but drastically lessened or even eradicated with just one precise treatment.

This chapter laid the groundwork for how gene therapy can be an advanced technique of rewiring anxiety at its molecular level. Having learned about the importance of the 5-HT2A receptor in anxiety and the shortcomings of traditional management measures such as SSRIs, you are now ready to understand the potential of focusing on this receptor. Let's build on this scientific base and look into the next-generation technologies. CRISPR and RNA therapeutics have the potential to shift the paradigm of anxiety and mental health treatments. We will delve deeper into the mechanisms of these gene therapy techniques and explore the significance of targeting this specific receptor in combating anxiety and memory impairments.

3

The Building Blocks of Anxiety

DNA, RNA & Proteins

Addiction injures in many ways, including the distortion or denial of events.

When I was thirteen, my mother worked with my stepdad and left me and my older sister for a week. Despite being left to our devices, we did well—no disasters, no emergencies. A month later, however, I was blamed for getting into a missing stash of marijuana.

This was as shocking as it was provoking. I did not even touch the stuff, let alone think of stealing it. I tried to defend myself, but nobody listened. I was called a liar, and for the next six months, I was under constant suspicion: daily accusations, being scolded, reprimanded, and reminded of the alleged theft.

The climax came when my stepdad presented me with a choice: admit to my made-up drug theft scheme or forfeit the eighth-grade class trip, one that I had eagerly anticipated and worked hard to raise funds for. So, the thirteen-year-old me took the fall for something I had not done, while my stepdad smirked smugly. Being blamed for something I did not do, along with my mother's silence, left me feeling completely deserted. (Why didn't she defend me? Why didn't she say, "Hey, maybe my child is not a drug lord?" Nope, not a word.)

This sense of helplessness, silence, and injustice sowed more seeds of anxiety.

As a child falsely accused, I did not understand that helplessness, guilt, and stress were not only psychological states; they altered the *actual chemistry* of my body. These experiences left an imprint at the most basic levels, affecting how my body and mind handled stress.

Anxiety, it turns out, is not just a "feeling." It is a physical condition rooted in our cells, driven by the interplay of **DNA, RNA, and proteins**—the very building blocks of life. In this chapter, I will describe how these molecular players affect the mechanisms that are involved in the *encoding of anxiety* in order to provide the link between emotional stress and the physiological processes that sustain it. This connection will help us understand an important question: How do our genes and cellular machinery turn life experiences into long-lasting anxiety?

ADVANCES IN RESEARCH

Advances in research offer a ray of hope for future personalized solutions to health problems. One promising avenue is gene therapy, which shows potential not only for life-threatening illnesses but also for mental health conditions, including anxiety. Grasping the intricate workings of this treatment method requires delving into the components of life: DNA, RNA, and proteins. These tiny molecules are crucial in understanding how our genetic makeup impacts our well-being and how selectively modifying them in the future might even restore equilibrium in individuals struggling with anxiety disorders and other neuropsychiatric conditions.

Let me state from the outset that gene therapy is complicated, which is one of the biggest hurdles to understanding its science. My company's platform, for example, is exceedingly complex and requires a fundamental understanding of the brain and the molecular underpinnings of how **Clustered Regularly Interspaced Short Palindromic Repeats (CRISPR)** can be used to treat disorders such as anxiety.

When presenting a complex neural-related topic, such as the action potential, I often tell students, "This is not rocket science—it is neuroscience!" A goal in writing this book is to break down the essential building blocks of gene therapy, making it easier to grasp how our technology functions and its promise in medicine.

To understand gene editing, it helps to learn about key parts of a cell, like the nucleus (where DNA is stored) and the plasma membrane (which controls what goes in and out of the cell). While many may be familiar with the terms DNA and RNA, the differences in how CRISPR and **RNA interference (RNAi)** impact these essential molecules in the cell are less understood. CRISPR *directly modifies* DNA, whereas RNAi targets RNA. Therefore, by the end of this chapter, we'll be able to distinguish between these two molecules and their roles.

OVERVIEW OF THE CELL

The **cell** is the smallest unit of life, defined by its ability to sense and respond to its environment, undergo metabolism, and have heritable instructions in its DNA, giving it the potential to reproduce. Humans are multicellular organisms made up of roughly 35 trillion cells. I prefer to give context to big or small numbers, so in this manner, "How big is 35 trillion? This number translates to a stack of $1,000 bills 68 miles high!"

Importantly, not all cells are alike and can vary enormously in appearance and function. Despite these differences, all cells share common characteristics. In this model, the analogy I like to use is to consider the cell as a factory.

Figure 3.1 depicts the essential architecture of a cell, omitting many details for simplicity. A defining feature of every cell is the presence of a semi-permeable **plasma** membrane. This membrane has two layers: the outer layers co-mingle with water-based fluids, while the middle layer comprises fats called lipids. This has important implications regarding what can enter and leave the cell. Anything dissolved in water (**hydrophilic substances**) cannot diffuse through the membrane. Think of Italian dressing sitting in your fridge. It is separated into two components: the oil and the water/vinegar. To use this dressing, you shake it vigorously before dousing your salad because, as we know, oil and water do not mix.

In the cell, anything hydrophilic, such as ions (K^+, Na^+, Ca^{2+}), proteins, DNA, or small chemical molecules such as neurotransmitters, cannot pass through this membrane, whose interior comprises lipids (fat). Therefore, the plasma membrane is considered **selectively permeable.**

Figure 3.1: Standard Features of All Cells

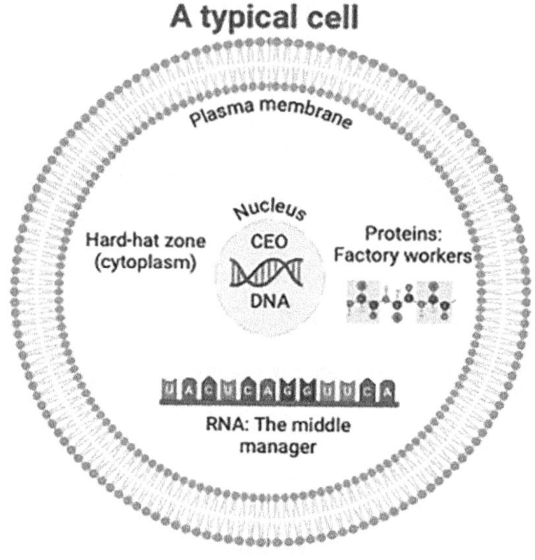

Note: The plasma membrane acts as a chain-linked fence, allowing tiny things to enter and exit, but larger hydrophilic substances cannot.

The "CEO's office," where the DNA, the "top manager," resides, is in the nucleus, and entry and exit are highly restrictive. The hard-hat zone is the cytoplasm where basic metabolism happens, and protein synthesis occurs under the "middle manager:" RNA.

DNA: The Top Managers

The leaders at the helm of our cells are the **genes**: the sections of DNA that oversee and guide all the functions within a cell's operations. These genes are inherited from our parents and serve as the blueprint for how the entire organism functions. DNA consists of strands of molecules known as nucleotides that are arranged to store information in a manner similar to words in a sentence.

This data leads to the production of **proteins**, which perform nearly all cell functions, from constructing cellular components like enzymes, transporters, and receptors to facilitating chemical reactions. In addition, proteins provide structure (such as collagen and elastin) and support to cells (like actin and microtubules), assist with cell communication (via hormones like insulin), and protect against health threats (such as antibodies).

Each gene functions similarly to a department within a vast organization. Some genes manage cell growth and division, while others supervise the creation of enzymes that facilitate metabolic activities in the body. Gene expression decides when and how much protein is made, which is crucial for keeping cells working properly.

Issues can arise from "mismanagement," like **mutations** or mistakes in the DNA sequence. These issues may result in conditions (such as anxiety disorder) that gene therapy seeks to treat.

In this way, DNA is like the assembly and instruction manual for life: full of cryptic instructions and missing screws that you might only discover when the anxiety kicks in. Genes contain the complete blueprints, creating and managing the cell's team of proteins for its functioning and upkeep. Without the blueprints in place, the vitality of life would be compromised.

RNA: The Middle Managers

The DNA acts as CEO in charge of the cell's function and growth blueprint, and it remains inside the nucleus, which serves as the central headquarters of cell operations.

Messenger RNA (**mRNA**) communicates and executes instructions to carry out tasks within the cell. This mRNA is an intermediary, dispatching the information from DNA to the hard-hat zone for protein synthesis. It differs from DNA's structure because it is a single-stranded molecule rather than the double-helix form of DNA. Its primary function is to replicate a DNA sequence from a gene through transcription. In essence, mRNA acts as a manager by conveying information from DNA to the operatives for creating proteins.

The creation of mRNA is closely monitored, much as middle managers oversee the distribution of instructions to their teams in a company setting. Not every gene undergoes transcription into mRNA continuously, as cells meticulously manage the activation and deactivation of genes based on the organism's requirements. This precise transcription process guarantees that only vital proteins are synthesized at a moment's notice to uphold the cell's functionality and harmony.

When the mRNA arrives at the **ribosomes** (the protein factories of all cells), it goes through a process known as translation. This process involves reading the mRNA's sequence of nucleotides and then utilizing it to arrange amino acids in the sequence to create a protein. The resulting protein can repair injuries, build structures, and transmit signals between cells.

In this context, mRNA conveys information and plays a crucial role in overseeing the cells' manufacturing process, guaranteeing that the correct proteins are synthesized when needed. First, the information in DNA is copied into mRNA during a process called transcription. The next step is translation, whereby the mRNA is read in groups of three nucleotides, known as codons, to form a protein. Note the use of linguistic terms: translation suggests a different language, for example, from English to French. In this case, the cell is translating from the nucleic acid language to the protein language.

Like a middle manager in a company setting up shop for a short stint before moving on to the next task at hand, mRNA plays a similar role in delivering its important instructions within our cells before being broken down and repurposed by the cells' recycling system. This avoids unnecessary protein production overload; the careful balance of regulation helps maintain harmony and efficiency within the cell's operations. However, when this process malfunctions or goes off track unexpectedly, it can result in issues like cancer or other diseases arising from protein levels being either too high or too low.

Overall, mRNA acts as a supervisor, ensuring that the cell effectively executes the commands from the DNA. Without these overseers, the vital transfer of information from the nucleus to the cytoplasm would be disrupted, bringing the cell and life's operations to a standstill.

This entire process of going from DNA>RNA>Protein is called the Central Dogma of Molecular Biology (Figure 3.2). (Frankly, this is an ugly, clunky term, and I am still determining where it originated. In school, we were taught that this process was called gene expression, which is more poetic!) Essentially, it refers to the flow of information that starts with DNA and ends with proteins. A critical result of gene expression is that cells can display differences in their structure and capabilities based on the genes that are active within them.

Figure 3.2: Gene Expression in All Cells

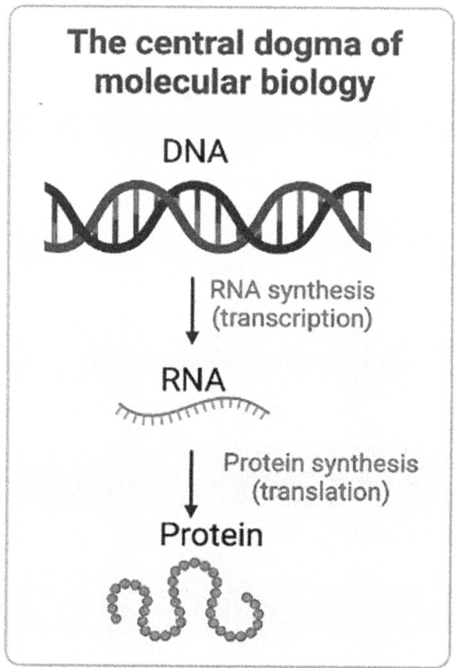

Note: The instructions in the DNA are read out (transcribed) and converted into mRNA. The message carried by the RNA molecule is converted (translated) into a protein molecule by linking amino acids.

This process serves as the core method by which stem cells transform into cell varieties, such as liver cells or **neurons**. For example, when a precursor cell develops into a liver cell, it explicitly activates genes for liver function, creating proteins essential for its functions.

When a stem cell becomes a liver cell, it then selectively expresses only the genes necessary for liver function, producing the specific proteins required for this role.

Neurons also exhibit this behavior by selectively expressing genes crucial for their role, such as voltage-gated ion channels, while disregarding others not needed for their function despite having the same complete set of genes shared by all cells.

A good analogy to understand this concept is considering a building manual for birdhouses. Each chapter comprises precise instructions on how to build a specific type of birdhouse. If you intended to make a bluebird house, you would only read that chapter, not other chapters, about creating a wren or woodpecker house. Cells behave similarly by adhering to the genetic "guidance" of their designated function; this enables them to specialize and carry out tasks while disregarding genetic information that is unnecessary for their responsibilities.

THE DIFFERENCE BETWEEN DNA & RNA

To fully appreciate gene therapy in the forthcoming chapters, it is essential to understand the difference between these two different types of nucleic acids. In addition to their structural and functional differences, another critical distinction between DNA and RNA is that they use different **nitrogenous bases**. While both molecules contain four of these bases, RNA uses uracil

(U) instead of thymine (T), which is found in DNA. In DNA, adenine pairs with thymine, but in RNA, adenine pairs with uracil. This difference contributes to each molecule's distinct roles in the cell (see Figure 3.3).

Another critical difference is the **half-life** of RNA compared to DNA. DNA is highly stable and designed to last for long periods, preserving and storing genetic information over the lifespan of an organism. RNA, however, is more unstable and has a shorter half-life, meaning it degrades more quickly. This short half-life allows RNA to be used for temporary tasks, such as synthesizing proteins, where it can be created, used, and broken down once it has served its purpose. Depending on the type of RNA, its half-life can range from minutes to a few hours, whereas DNA remains intact for a much more extended period.

Figure 3.3: Key Differences Between DNA & RNA

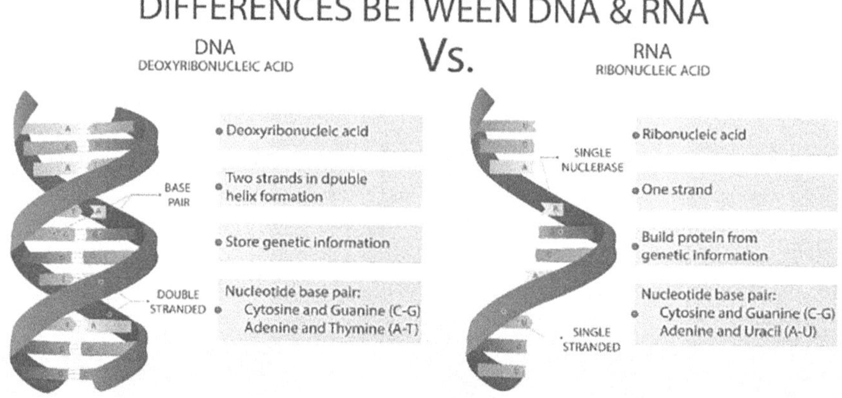

Note: DNA is double-stranded, forming a twisted helix structure, and its central role is to store genetic information. It uses the nucleotide base pairs adenine (A) with thymine (T) and cytosine (C) with guanine (G). In contrast, RNA is single stranded and helps in protein synthesis by translating genetic information from DNA into proteins. RNA's nucleotide base pairs include adenine (A) with uracil (U) and cytosine (C) with guanine (G). Adapted from Shutterstock.com.

DNA and RNA are both key players in gene therapy processes; however, the resulting proteins also support cellular functions, effectively completing the picture of gene therapy. DNA acts as the blueprint, and RNA acts as the messenger. Meanwhile, proteins function as laborers, carrying out various cell tasks ranging from providing structure to facilitating cell reactions and communication. As when forming different types of cells, when a gene is activated and put into action in the body's system of processes and functions, the protein performs the task as directed by the DNA blueprint of instructions within cells. Proteins serve roles such as catalyst enzymes that accelerate biochemical reactions in living organisms.

Proteins can also serve as receptors that facilitate communication between cells or structural elements, such as actin, that provide cells with their characteristic structure and ability to move (Figure 3.4).

The primary goal of gene therapy frequently involves repairing DNA to restore proper protein function. By altering or adjusting the information encoded in our DNA, the cells can adjust and control the creation of specific proteins, determine their quantity, and potentially rectify any faulty versions. Another helpful analogy: Proteins are the overworked interns of the cell. DNA is the micromanaging boss sending out instructions via the RNA, and proteins run around doing everything, such as building the walls, fixing communication systems, or cleaning up biochemical messes. Gene therapy? That is HR stepping in to rewrite the job descriptions from headquarters so that the interns stop making catastrophic mistakes!

Now, what do functional proteins do?

Figure 3.4: Six Key Roles that Proteins Play in the Cell Membrane

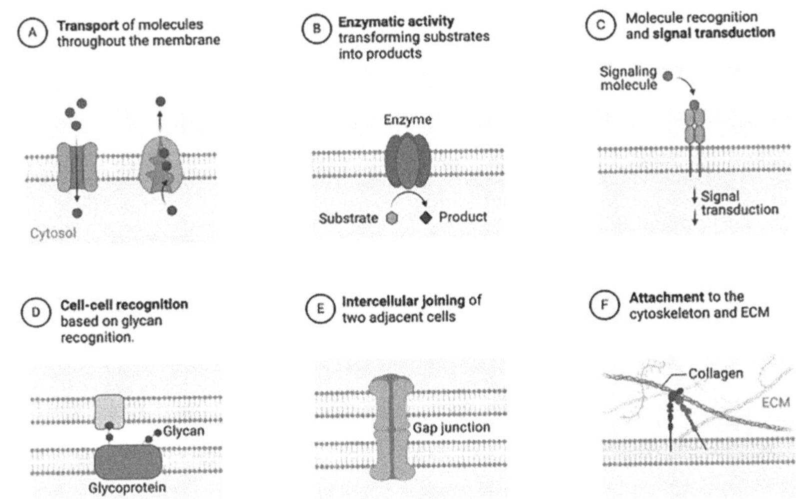

The six key roles depicted in Figure 3.4 are:

- **Transport:** Proteins help move molecules like nutrients or ions into and out of the cell.
- **Enzymatic activity:** Some proteins act as enzymes, speeding up chemical reactions inside or outside the cell.
- **Signal recognition and transduction:** Membrane proteins can detect signals outside the cell and trigger responses inside.
- **Cell to cell recognition:** Proteins help cells recognize each other, which is essential for communication and immune responses.
- **Intercellular joining:** Proteins allow cells to connect and work together as a unit.
- **Attachment to the cytoskeleton and extracellular matrix:** Some proteins anchor the cell to its surroundings and help maintain its shape.

To summarize, gene expression is the process of synthesizing proteins from genes. It starts when a specific gene needs to be expressed, and the segment of DNA containing this gene is transcribed into messenger RNA (mRNA). The mRNA then leaves the nucleus and travels to the **ribosome** for protein synthesis, where amino acids are linked together to form a polypeptide.

This process is crucial to life and shows the possibility of gene therapy. In modifying DNA, we can control the synthesis of proteins and thus address the problems that cause diseases. For instance, some anxiety disorders *may* be a result of genetic variations that affect the synthesis of important proteins, such as the 5-HT2A receptor that is involved in the regulation of mood. For instance, research has demonstrated that specific single-nucleotide polymorphisms (SNPs) in the *HTR2A* gene, which encodes the 5-HT2A receptor, are associated with panic disorder and other anxiety disorders, such as social anxiety disorder (Vermeire et al., 2009; Unschuld et al., 2007). This indicates a genetic basis for altered serotonergic signaling in those suffering from anxiety, underscoring the importance of the 5-HT2A receptor in these conditions.

In this chapter, I described life's molecular components, including DNA, RNA, and proteins, and the process of gene expression. Changes in genes, such as those that code for neurotransmitter receptors, can lead to changes in protein function and thus could lead to anxiety.

Through altering the information in the DNA or RNA, it's hoped that gene therapy can be used to balance the proteins, their impacts, and the resulting bodily systems. This capability provides the possibility for a new and more accurate therapeutic strategy for anxiety and other neuropsychiatric disorders.

4

From Code To Chaos

How DNA Shapes Brain Chemistry & Anxiety

Being subjected to repeated stress is part of developing PTSD. This stress, in my case, included being blamed and shamed.

In my sophomore year of high school, history repeated itself when my stepdad accused me of stealing money. After several months of verbal abuse, he made me an outrageous offer: take a lie detector test, and if I failed, well, punishment would be forthcoming.

Weeks later, having called his bluff, I had wires strapped to my body, feeling more like a criminal than a kid. I kept thinking: Who the hell does this to their child? I was terrified—my heart raced, and my mind played out every possible scenario where my fear would betray me and I would fail, regardless of the truth. Somehow, despite my anxious state, I passed the test with flying colors.

The injustice of having to validate my innocence in such an absurd and humiliating way became a silent cornerstone of the anxiety I would battle for years to come.

The trauma of being unfairly accused and the resulting mental wounds it left behind (today, this is often referred to as "moral injury") taught me a profound lesson: the damage caused by unresolved problems can fester, affecting every aspect of life. Whether it is family dynamic problems or a genetic mutation within the body, addressing the source of an issue is the only way to truly heal. This is the promise of gene therapy: a chance to confront illnesses at their foundation, correcting the very instructions that lead to disease.

Yet, *can* anxiety be treated with gene therapy? We have recently entered a new medical era, moving towards better disease treatment strategies with a single gene therapy session. This idea is no longer pie-in-the-sky but a reality.

Sickle cell disease is a genetic disorder affecting millions of people globally and is caused by a mutation in a gene responsible for the production of hemoglobin in the body. Unlike the standard concave shape that red blood cells should have, in sickle cell disease, cells become stiff and take on a crescent form resembling a sickle. These shaped cells can obstruct blood vessels, leading to blockages in blood flow and resulting in severe pain and severe long-term complications (Tanabe et al., 2019).

Standard treatments have focused on symptom management. While bone marrow or stem cell transplants have been considered a cure in some cases, they come with significant risks and challenges related to finding donors. Despite these treatment options, individuals with sickle cell disease have often encountered health struggles and a shortened lifespan.

The recent U.S. Food and Drug Administration (FDA) approval of a CRISPR-based gene therapy (called **Casgevy**) (US Food and Drug Administration, 2023) has sparked hope for those affected by this condition. CRISPR is a technology that enables scientists to modify specific genes, offering the promise of curing sickle cell disease by targeting the underlying genetic mutation. Patients involved in trials of CRISPR gene therapy have shown improvements in symptoms that subside or disappear entirely (US Food and Drug Administration, 2023).

Understanding the protein-making process in cells is essential for grasping the transformative benefits of CRISPR gene therapy.

THE ATCGS OF MAKING A PROTEIN

To understand how CRISPR works, it is essential to know how DNA leads to the production of a specific protein. Both CRISPR and RNAi aim to regulate protein production. Proteins are the ultimate products of gene expression and play critical roles in various processes, from muscle movement to brain function.

Just as the page you are reading contains letters arranged in discrete information units known as words, and those words combine to create sentences, paragraphs, and chapters, DNA contains nucleotides arranged into genes and then chromosomes. Again, we can think of DNA as a blueprint that contains all the information regarding the construction of a particular cell molecule. The materials it uses are just four bases: Adenine (A), Guanine (G), Cytosine (C), and Thymine (T). These letters pair up so that A always pairs with T while G always pairs with C, combining to form the DNA structure in the form of a twisted ladder.

When a cell requires a protein, it first requires a specific part of the DNA to be transcribed into a molecule called mRNA, which (as we read earlier) works as the middle manager for the DNA. The mRNA carries the message out of the DNA's "control center" (the nucleus) to the part of the cell where proteins are made. The mRNA provides the order in which the building blocks of proteins and amino acids should be connected.

The message is read in groups of three "letters," called codons. For example, the mRNA codon AUG signals the start of a protein and codes for the amino acid methionine.

Figure 4.1: Using DNA to Create Proteins

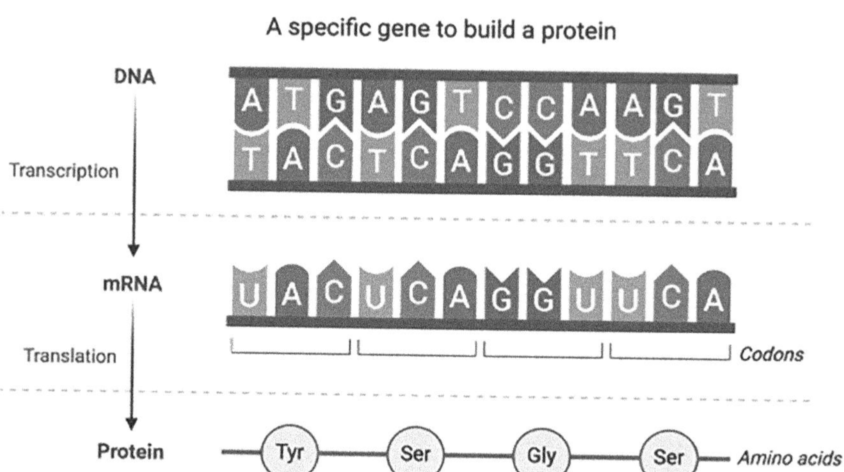

Note: This schematic illustrates the process of using DNA to create proteins. First, the information in DNA is copied into mRNA during a process called transcription. The next step is translation, whereby the mRNA is read in groups of three nucleotides, known as codons, to form a protein. Each codon represents an amino acid.

Some codons signal the cell to stop building the protein once it is complete. This process is how your DNA instructions are turned into the proteins your body needs to function (Figure 4.1). Also, three codons, UAG, UGA, and UAA, do not specify amino acids but act as termination signals (or punctuation) in the protein translation process. When any of these stop codons are encountered within an mRNA strand, the synthesis of the corresponding protein is finished.

Think of mRNA as the cell's overenthusiastic project manager: it grabs the instructions from DNA, rushes out of the nucleus like it is late for a meeting, and hands them off to the ribosome, saying,

"Here, follow these specs exactly!" And when it hits a "stop" codon? That is the protein's cue to drop its tools and clock out.

MUTATIONS: CHANGES IN THE DNA SEQUENCE

The specific order of codons in mRNA plays an essential role in ensuring the amino acids are correctly added in the precise order of the growing protein chain. Every protein will always have the same DNA and RNA sequence, as well as the same number and sequence of amino acids. For example, the enzyme lysozyme (found in tears and kills bacteria) will always have 129 amino acids in the same order from start to finish.

However, when a **mutation** either adds or takes away DNA bases (also called nucleotides), it can completely alter how these codons are read. This kind of mutation is called a **frameshift mutation**. It changes how the genetic code is interpreted and the resulting lineup of amino acids.

Consequently, the resulting protein might not function properly, leading to disease, as occurs with the protein hemoglobin in sickle cell disease. Even more damage occurs when frameshift mutations lead to the introduction of a premature stop codon early in the mRNA coding sequence. This leads to a truncated protein that (inevitably) is quickly destroyed by the cell (Figure 4.2).

Figure 4.2: DNA Mutations Can Affect the mRNA Sequence

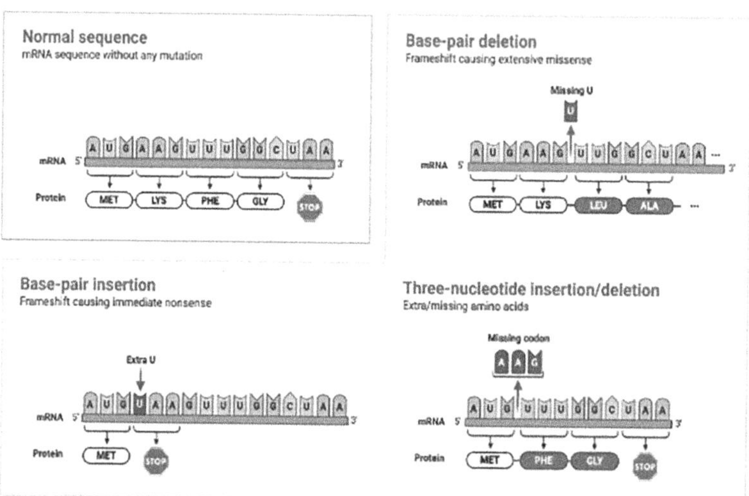

Note: This figure illustrates how different DNA mutations can affect the mRNA sequence and the resulting protein. The normal sequence in the top-left panel shows an mRNA sequence with no mutations, producing a functional protein. In the top-right panel, a base-pair deletion removes a single base/nucleotide, causing a "frameshift mutation." This mutation alters the reading frame and changes the resulting amino acids. The bottom-left panel shows a base-pair insertion, where an extra nucleotide causes an immediate stop codon, leading to a shortened, nonfunctional protein. Finally, the bottom-right panel shows a three-nucleotide insertion/deletion, which removes or adds a whole codon, leading to the loss or addition of an amino acid without shifting the reading frame. However, the missing codon still affects the protein structure.

In addition to potentially introducing a premature stop codon, another consequence is a change in the **reading frame**. The insertion or deletion of nucleotides changes the reading frame, meaning the following codons are shifted and misinterpreted. When this happens, the protein ends up with the wrong amino acids, making the protein unable to fold correctly and carry out its function.

Tay-Sachs disease is an example of a frameshift disorder seen in the nervous system. This frameshift mutation occurs in the *HEX* gene, resulting in a faulty protein that cannot properly break down fatty compounds in the brain and nerve cells. In this disease, the mutation alters the reading frame, resulting in a protein with an incorrect sequence of amino acids. The misshapen protein no longer has the proper structure or function, leading to the buildup of fatty substances in the brain and to the symptoms linked to this fatal neurological disease (Figure 4.3).

Figure 4.3: A Frameshift Mutation Leads to Tay-Sachs Disease

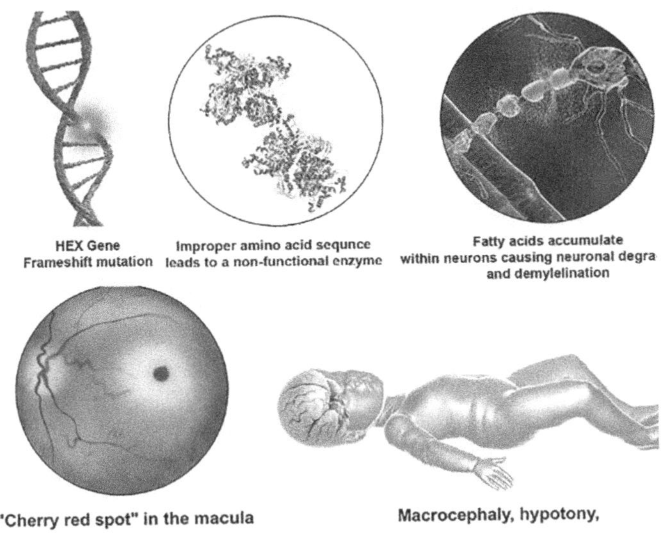

Note: Mutations in the HEXA gene lead to a nonfunctional enzyme (hexosaminidase A) that is quickly degraded by the neuronal cells. Because this enzyme is supposed to break down certain fatty substances called gangliosides, accumulating these fats leads to eventual neuronal death, loss of motor skills and vision, seizures, and eventually other problems. Unfortunately,

children with Tay-Sachs do not live beyond early childhood. Adapted from Kateryna Kon/Shutterstock.com.

An, additional illustration of a frameshift disorder is Duchenne muscular dystrophy (DMD). This mutation is passed down through a recessive inheritance pattern, resulting in the progressive deterioration of skeletal muscle tissues. This disorder is transmitted as an X-linked trait, and because males only carry a single X chromosome, this disorder exclusively affects males.

The gene in question is referred to as the dystrophin gene. The expression of this gene leads to a protein known as dystrophin, which serves a crucial function in maintaining the stability of muscle cell membranes during their contraction process. When a frameshift mutation occurs, it causes the generation of an ineffective, severely truncated form of dystrophin that quickly becomes degraded. Consequently, this results in muscle cells' progressive weakening and death (Figure 4.4).

Figure 4.4: Duchenne's Muscular Dystrophy (DMD)

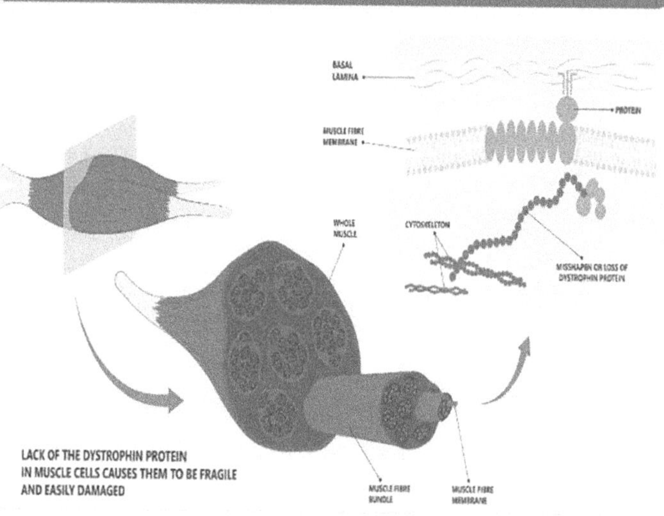

Note: The dystrophin protein plays a role in upholding the integrity of muscle cells. When it is absent or malfunctioning, as depicted, muscle fibers become delicate and prone to damage. Insufficient functional dystrophin causes muscle cells to struggle with the high mechanical demands of activities, resulting in a breakdown of muscle tissue over time.

Signs of Duchenne dystrophy typically manifest during childhood, between the ages of three and five years old, with initial weakness in the leg and pelvic muscles observed in affected children. Children with DMD commonly encounter challenges engaging in activities such as running and climbing stairs due to muscle weakness. As the condition advances, it impacts muscles throughout the body, resulting in mobility issues, with some children losing their walking ability by age twelve. Eventually, the loss of functional dystrophin and subsequent breakdown of skeletal muscle impacts breathing and heart functions. The mean age of death is between ages sixteen and twenty-four and occurs as a result of respiratory failure, cardiac complications, congestive heart failure, and arrhythmias.

How does the frameshift mutation in the dystrophin gene lead to the failure of dystrophin protein production? A mutation in the dystrophin gene alters the dystrophin RNA so that it no longer codes for functional dystrophin protein, usually due to a mutation that alters the reading frame.

To fully understand the frameshift mutation in the dystrophin gene, we need to understand another concept: the difference between an **exon** and an **intron** in the DNA genome. A gene can be compared to a recipe for making a protein. It contains instructions on how to create a specific dish (exons) necessary for protein creation. The introns lie between the exons and serve as notes or comments in the recipe that are not essential to the actual content of the dish protein-making process.

When a cell interprets the instructions to produce a protein molecule, the cells *discard* the introns and retain only the functional regions called exons. This might be analogous to skimming unnecessary footnotes in a recipe and concentrating solely on the essential cooking directions.

A gene contains the introns and exons; the pre-RNA transcript also harbors both. A process known as **splicing** cuts out the introns, and the subsequent exons are pasted together. This final product produces the mature form of mRNA, which is then translated into protein.

Think of a gene as a sentence where every three letters form a word like "THE CAT ATE RAT." In cases of DMD, occasionally, a letter (symbolizing part of the genetic code) gets inserted or deleted, causing all the following parts to shift. For instance, if you eliminate the 'H' in 'THE,' the sentence now reads 'TE CAT ATE RAT,' losing its meaning altogether. As discussed, this is precisely what occurs in Tay-Sachs disease.

In DMD, this mutation goes beyond a mere loss of a single letter—it can result in the loss of one entire exon (or even multiple exons), which are vital components of the gene structure itself. When these exons are missing from the gene sequence, the cell encounters difficulties accurately interpreting the instructions for producing the dystrophin protein. The outcome is a protein that's either too short, deficient, or outright nonfunctional, resulting in muscle weakness and deterioration.

Unlike other conditions that can be improved with treatments like physical therapy, corticosteroids, or newer gene therapies to alleviate symptoms, DMD remains challenging to cure and requires more comprehensive management to enhance the well-being of those affected. Recent progress in gene editing tools like CRISPR and RNA interference has sparked optimism for interventions to address the fundamental genetic abnormalities linked to DMD (Figure 4.5).

Figure 4.5: Impact of Alterations in the Dystrophin Gene

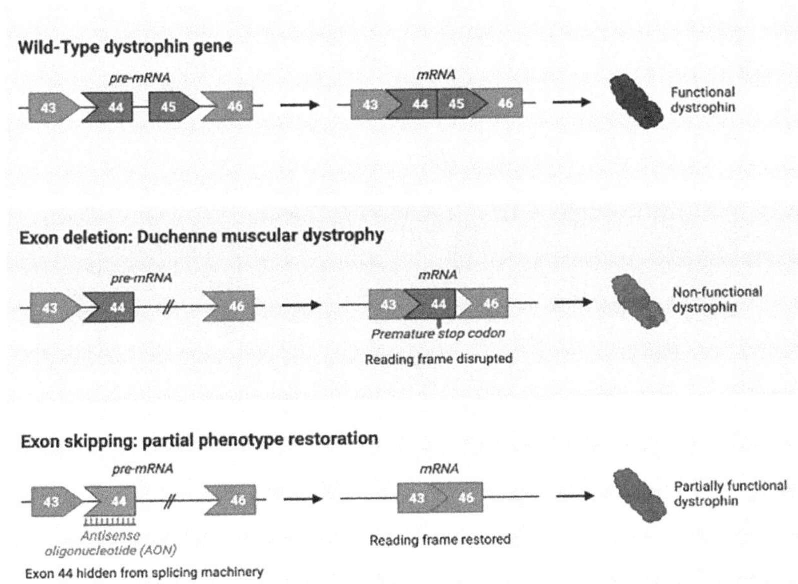

Note: Exons 43–46 are accurately connected to form the functional dystrophin protein. In DMD, a deletion results in the loss of exon 45 within the gene sequence, which disrupts the gene's reading frame, triggering an early stop signal and producing a truncated non-functional protein. Exon-skipping therapy involves a method where exon 44 is concealed from the genes reading mechanism, which allows exons 43 and 46 to join, skipping the faulty exon and restoring part of the reading frame. Consequently, a shorter yet partly operable dystrophin protein is manufactured. This process is the basis for the FDA-approved drug Casimersen (brand name Amondys 45), currently used as a new treatment for DMD.

The examples detailed in this chapter demonstrate that gene expression is a complex process, one that can be significantly affected by minor molecular alterations in the DNA. DMD is just one compelling example of how genetic mutations that lead to frameshift mutations can have devastating effects on the protein synthesis process and cause disease.

However, new techniques provide hope in the form of gene therapy that is not only limited to rare diseases such as DMD but also to more common conditions, including anxiety. Gene therapy can alter imbalances in genetic coding and provide new forms of treatment. As we gain knowledge of the genetic code and its relation to various conditions, we can envision the possibilities for personal, tailored treatments for those affected by life-threatening diseases.

Part II

Engineering Calm Through Gene Editing & Ethical Innovation

5

Rewriting the Blueprint

How CRISPR Offers New Hope for Anxiety Sufferers

Anxiety manifests in my day-to-day life in very subtle ways, not in fear or trepidation, but in my interactions with other people. To be blunt, I often dislike being around human beings. More than just occasionally feeling shy, I am, by nature, a loner, and when I have to be put in social situations, especially with strangers, it makes me feel very uncomfortable. Small talk with others is draining, much like depleting the battery of an iPhone.

Even worse is speaking on that iPhone! Today, though, I can joke with my wife and kids that I have been struck with the "Rohn" gene.

My wife is utterly perplexed by this behavior and understandably becomes frustrated. Moreover, if I cannot bring my wife along, I'd at least settle for my service dog, Bailey! My favorite stickers on my Hydro Flask are, "The best therapist has fur and four legs" and "Dog Friendly. Human Selective."

I have learned to recognize some of the symptoms of anxiety (as outlined by HelpGuide.org):

- Excessive self-consciousness and anxiety in everyday social situations

- Intense worry for days, weeks, or even months before an upcoming social situation
- Avoiding social situations to a degree that limits your activities or disrupts your life
- Staying quiet or hiding in the background to escape notice
- Needing to bring a buddy wherever you go

This type of anxiety is a part of me, and, joking aside, I feel like it is in my genes. However, what if it could be different? What if the genetic and molecular mechanisms that are associated with anxiety could be modified or even overridden, changing the program that leads to such anxiety? This is where CRISPR technology provides new hope.

WHAT IS CRISPR?

CRISPR/Cas9 has given scientists the capacity to alter the genes that define anxiety, which means that one can now treat the problem at its core. In this chapter, I will first explain what CRISPR is and how it works, and then discuss why it is such a hopeful tool for the treatment of anxiety and how it could one day improve the lives of those who suffer from more than just "nerves."

The discovery of CRISPR is a story that unfolded over many years, originating in a puzzling find within the DNA of bacteria. The double-helix structure having been revealed many years earlier, in 1987, Japanese scientists found sequences of genetic material that repeated regularly, with unique DNA segments between them.

During that time, the significance of these sequences remained a mystery.

No one could have foreseen how that seemingly trivial observation would reshape the field of biology. In 2002, scientists finally assigned a name to the DNA patterns they observed: **Clustered Regularly**

Interspaced Short Palindromic Repeats (CRISPR). These sequences were found not in one type of bacteria but across various species.

Despite this discovery, the purpose of CRISPR remained a mystery. What exactly was the role of these DNA sequences? Why were they so prevalent? In the mid-2000s came the revelation that CRISPR was a component of a bacterial defense mechanism against viruses (yes, even bacteria are regularly under attack from these little pests!). When a *virus* infects a bacterium, it leaves its mark as a snippet of DNA, which is then captured within the CRISPR segment of the *bacterium's* makeup. Upon any subsequent invasion by the same virus threat, the bacterium can promptly identify and neutralize it by exploiting this stored genetic information. Thus, CRISPR essentially acts like a memory for bacteria, enabling them to recall viral infections and quickly defend themselves against future invasions.

Another turning point in the field came in 2012, when seminal research by Jennifer Doudna and Emmanuelle Charpentier uncovered the potential of utilizing this bacterial defense mechanism for genetic editing. They pinpointed a protein called **Cas9**, which acts as molecular scissors to precisely sever DNA strands at designated sites. By creating a **guide RNA** based on the CRISPR system, scientists could direct Cas9 towards any part of the entire DNA genome, opening up the possibility of a new gene editing mechanism (Jinek et al., 2012). This breakthrough revolutionized the field of biology, and for their discovery, Doudna and Charpentier were awarded the Nobel Prize in Chemistry in 2020.

The CRISPR/Cas9 system rapidly emerged as a new tool to enable geneticists and medical researchers to edit parts of the genome by removing, adding, or altering sections of the DNA genome. It is currently the most straightforward, versatile, and precise method of genetic manipulation, and dozens of clinical trials are already underway to harness the potential of CRISPR in treating numerous diseases and disorders (Table 5.1).

Table 5.1: A Partial List of CRISPR Therapeutics in Clinical Development

COMPANY	TREATMENT	INDICATION	STATUS
CRISPR Therapeutics/ Vertex Pharmaceuticals	Exa-cel	Sickle cell disease/ Transfusion dependent beta thalassemia	FDA approval, December 2023
Editas Medicine	EDIT-301	Sickle cell disease	Phase I/II trial
Graphite Bio	Nula-cel	Sickle cell disease	Phase I/II trial
Intellia Therapeutics	NTLA-2002	Hereditary angioedema	Phase III trial
CRISPR Therapeutics	CTX310	Cardiovascular disease	Phase II trial

Note: These studies are ongoing for all therapeutics listed in the "Status" column. (Source: GlobalData, Clinicaltrials.gov, and private company updates).

THE MECHANICS OF CRISPR

CRISPR allows scientists to edit DNA, similar to programming a computer. This technique significantly enhances the speed, ease, cost, and accuracy of DNA editing. The potential impact of this technology on human civilization has even been compared to transformative innovations like the steam engine and the transistor.

The CRISPR system has two major components: the guide RNA and the Cas9 protein (see Figure 5.1).

Figure 5.1: Two Key Components of CRISPR

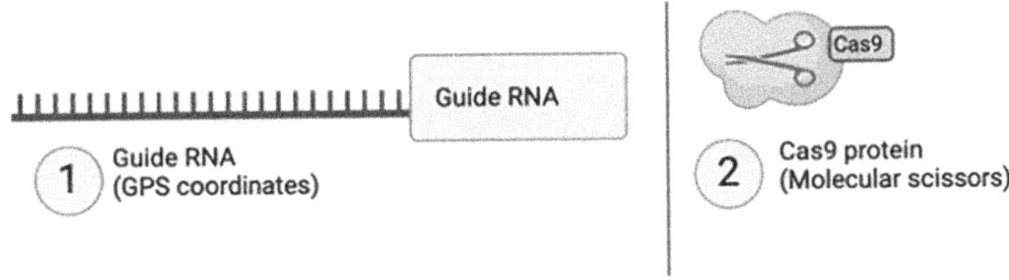

Note: The guide RNA acts like a set of GPS coordinates, directing the Cas9 protein to the precise location in the DNA that needs to be altered. Once at the target, the Cas9 protein functions as molecular scissors, cutting both DNA strands of the helix to enable the desired changes.

The accurate and successful editing of genes using CRISPR heavily relies on the **guide RNA** (gRNA) design. Think of the gRNA as the GPS coordinates for the Cas9 protein in the DNA landscape known as the genome.

Consider that the genome contains 3 x 10^9 base pairs (nucleotides). How significant is this number? If you were to hire a typist who can type 60 words/minute, eight hours a day, it would take more than 50 years to type out 3 x 10^9 base pairs! It is not an overstatement to say that the ability of the gRNA to find the correct sequence is like finding a needle in a haystack.

Furthermore, there is a limit to the length of the gRNA, typically set at around 20 nucleotides. It is critical to ensure that a 20-base-pair sequence is unique to only the gene of interest among the 3 x 10^9 base pairs. Otherwise, unintended cuts in the DNA by Cas9 could lead to *serious* off-target effects, including unintended gene disruption, altered cell function, and therapeutic risks.

Fortunately, scientists have tools to predict potential off-target cuts using *in silico* online algorithms. One of my favorite algorithms, for example, is CHOPCHOP. This tool allows researchers to input the gene of interest, where the program will spit out the top 100 gRNA sequences as well as data for each sequence, including the predicted off-target cut sites.

Access to such tools is critical to research and treatment. The success and safety of CRISPR-based treatments greatly hinge on the quality of gRNA design. Again, a misaligned cut could interfere with genes or regulatory parts, resulting in catastrophic consequences.

THE IMPACT OF CRISPR ON GENE EXPRESSION

How do gRNA and Cas9 work together to silence gene expression?

The key to understanding this process is recognizing that all cells possess DNA repair mechanisms essential for minimizing the occurrence of mutations. Mutations may occur through normal DNA replication as cells divide or through environmental insults that can alter the DNA directly, including ultraviolet light and chemical carcinogens.

DNA has two systems for fixing breaks in cells. **Homology-directed repair (HDR)** and **non-homologous end joining (NHEJ)**.

HDR works like a repair tool that utilizes a matching section of DNA to mend the break precisely and accurately restore the DNA to its initial condition.

However, HDR can only occur in dividing cells because it depends on having a duplicate template present during cell division. Neurons, which are non-dividing cells, cannot utilize HDR for repairs and rely upon NHEJ to repair any breaks in the DNA strands.

Unlike HDR, which necessitates a template for mending DNA breaks, NHEJ directly reconnects the severed DNA ends without external guidance. Although this approach is quicker, it is also much less accurate. Sometimes, we refer to this as the "better-than-nothing" repair system.

This repair system is the last-resort mechanism to repair double-strand breaks in the DNA (Figure 5.2). NHEJ is a type of repair that occurs even in cells that cannot divide, such as neurons.

Consider the DNA as a ladder composed of countless rungs or steps. When there is damage, or when editing tools like CRISPR are used, the ladder can be damaged and snap into two. NHEJ acts as a rapid response repair crew that hurries in to mend the ladder. However, the repair work is usually sloppy and prone to including small mistakes.

Figure 5.2: Two Methods to Mend Double-Stranded Breaks (DSBs)

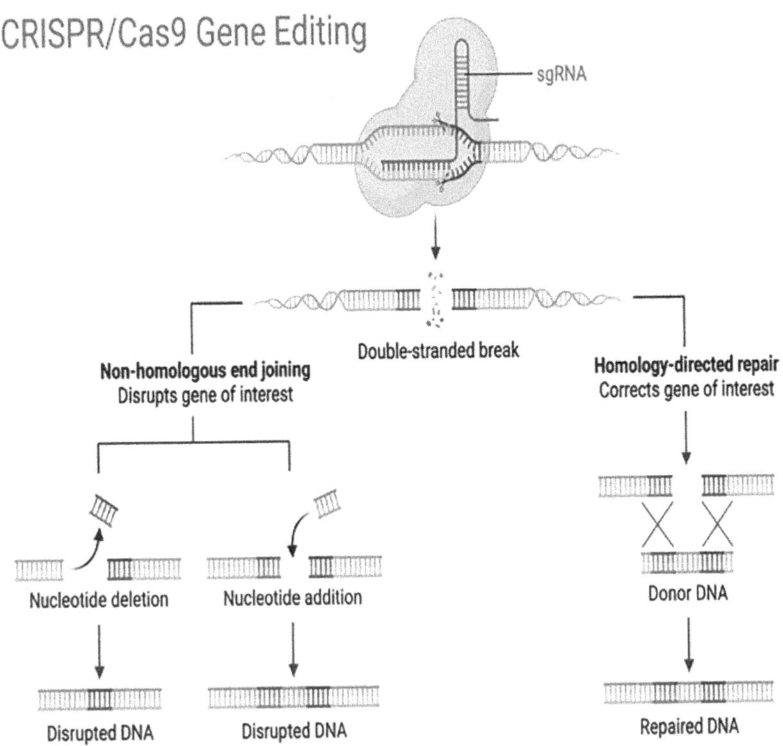

Note: Following cleavage by CRISPR/Cas9, two methods can mend the breaks. On the left is non-homologous end joining (NHEJ), a faster

but less accurate technique than HDR. The right side depicts homology-directed repair (HDR), which mends the break precisely. From Dragt, Esmée (Creator), & Ngai, Louis (2017). Using CRISPR in your experiments. In CRISPR 101: A Desktop Resource (pp. 30-93). Addgene.

Figure 5.2 also explains how CRISPR/Cas9 can lead to gene silencing.

Imagine DNA as a long instruction manual, where every sentence is carefully written to guide the cell's functions. When CRISPR/Cas9 creates a break in the DNA, the cell tries to fix it using NHEJ, which is like taping up a torn page. However, NHEJ often makes mistakes, like inserting random letters or deleting parts of a sentence.

These errors can change the meaning of the instructions, sometimes creating "nonsense" sentences that do not work anymore.

In gene silencing, however, this "nonsense" effect is helpful because it shuts down the gene completely. It's more like crossing out an entire section of the manual. Scientists *intentionally* use this error-prone method to turn off specific genes when they do not want them to function, making NHEJ a helpful tool for disrupting harmful genes (Rohn et al., 2018).

APPLICATIONS OF CRISPR TO TREAT ILLNESS: HUNTINGTON'S DISEASE & SICKLE CELL

A real-world illustration of this technology is seen in Huntington's Disease (HD), which causes neurodegeneration due to a mutation in the HTT gene. The HTT gene provides the instructions for creating the Huntington protein; however, scientists are not yet certain what function the protein performs. However, it's clear that HD results from genetic alterations that produce a defective form of this protein, which slowly destroys brain cells, particularly those involved in movement, thinking, and anxiety.

The effect of the HTT mutation is different from what occurs in DMD (discussed in an earlier chapter) in that it is a form of "repeat expansion" disorder. This means that a small piece of the gene's code—CAG—is duplicated *many* more times than it should be. In normal individuals, the CAG sequence is reiterated between 10 and 27 times, while in HD, it can vary from 40 to 120 times, resulting in toxic protein formation (Figure 5.3).

Figure 5.3: HD's Altered Versions of the Huntington Protein

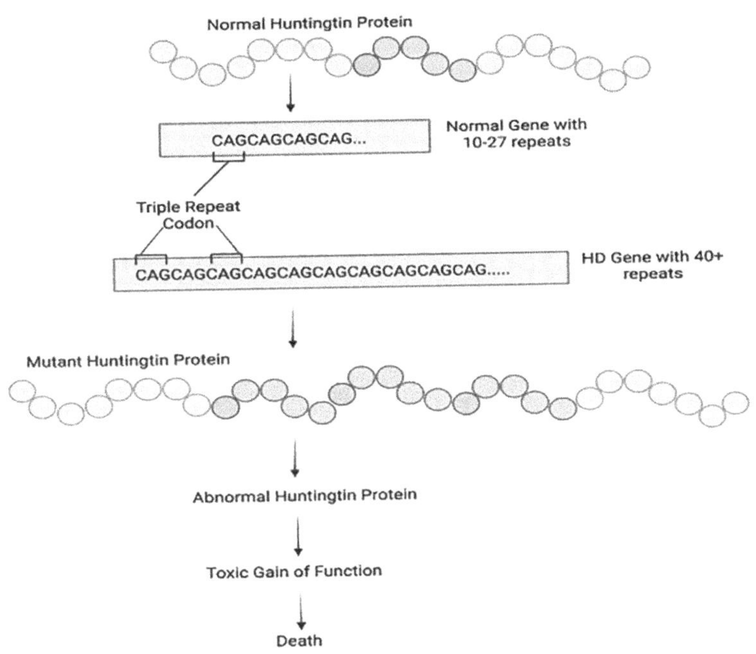

Note: The upper section displays the normal gene, with 10 to 27 CAG tri-nucleotides. In contrast, the lower section illustrates the HD gene, with 40 or more CAG repeats leading to a mutated form of the protein. The lower part

shows that the altered protein acquires a toxic gain of function and eventual neuron death, leading to the symptoms of HD.

Scientists believe that the corresponding increase in the total number of amino acids leads to a form of the protein that becomes toxic. As this toxic protein accumulates within neurons, it leads to neuronal death and symptoms of the disease. Currently, there is no treatment or cure for this devastating disorder. Think of the CAG repeat in Huntington's as a glitch in your phone's autocorrect: once is annoying, twice is frustrating, but 40 times?

Suddenly, you are typing gibberish, and everything crashes—except this time, the brain cells are throwing in the towel.

Scientists are exploring how CRISPR technology can target and modify the mutated *HTT* gene (Yang et al., 2017). One aim is to deactivate the gene employing CRISPR by making cuts at locations within its DNA sequence. This disruption hinders protein production, potentially slowing or stopping disease progression. In preclinical animal models, this approach has proven effective in mitigating the damaging effects of the toxic huntingtin protein (Yang et al., 2017). Clinical trials using CRISPR to treat HD are currently in the planning stages.

Chapter 4 discussed sickle cell disease, for which CRISPR was first approved. How does CRISPR work in this disease? To reiterate, sickle cell disease is caused by a mutation in the gene that encodes hemoglobin, a red blood cell protein responsible for transporting oxygen. This point mutation changes a single amino acid, leading to various symptoms associated with the disorder, including fatigue, dizziness, painful episodes, and vision problems. Sickle cell disease is a genetic disorder caused by mutations in hemoglobin genes. These mutations lead to a faulty hemoglobin protein called **hemoglobin S**. Hemoglobin S changes flexible red blood cells into rigid, sickle-shaped cells (Figure 5.4). As we've learned, sickled cells can block blood flow and cause pain and organ damage.

Figure 5.4: A Slight Alteration in DNA Results in Sickle Cell Disease

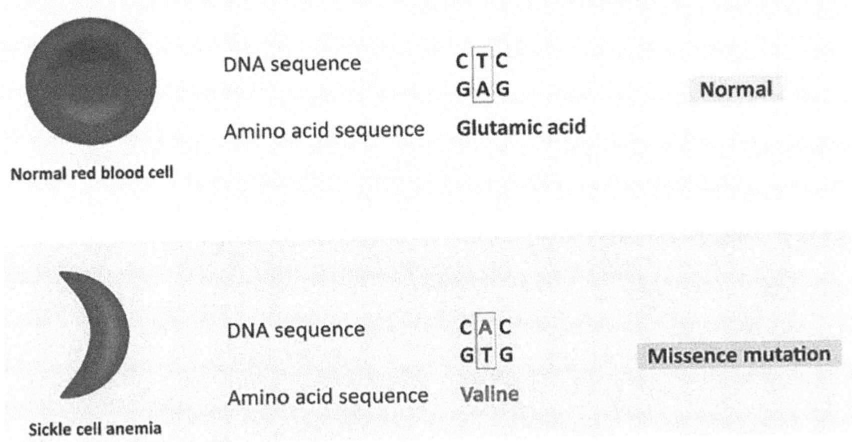

Note: In red blood cells (top), the genetic codon displays "CTC," which codes for the amino acid glutamic acid and maintains the round and pliable shape of the red blood cells. In sickle cell disease (bottom), a genetic mutation changes the DNA sequence to "CAC," resulting in valine being inserted as the amino acid. This small change alters the entire red blood cell structure into rigid red blood cells with a sickle-like shape; these cells can obstruct blood flow and lead to health issues.

CRISPR gene editing therapy, such as Casgevy (exa-cel), addresses sickle cell disease by focusing on the genetic defect that triggers the illness. Instead of directly repairing the sickle cell mutation, Casgevy *activates* a different gene that increases fetal hemoglobin production. This type of hemoglobin does not sickle. So, instead of knocking out a gene that produces a disease-causing protein, Casgevy targets a regulatory element to disrupt the normal repression of the fetal hemoglobin gene.

This process results in healthier red blood cells. The treatment includes gathering the patient's stem cells and modifying them with Casgevy externally before reinserting them into the patient's body (Figure 5.5). The improved cells will generate red blood cells that lessen sickling and alleviate symptoms. By boosting the quantity of red blood cells, Casgevy can significantly improve the patient's daily life and substantially minimize sickle cell disease complications.

Figure 5.5: Gene Therapy for Sickle Cell Disease

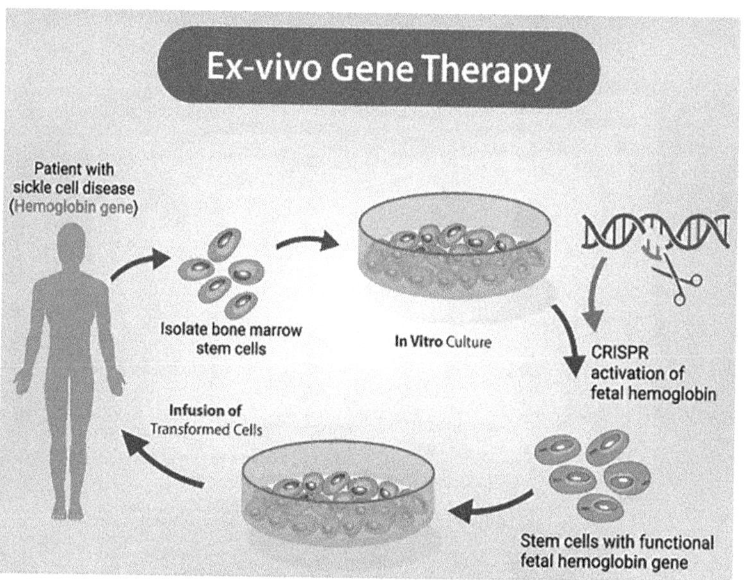

Note: Stem cells from a sickle cell disease patient are extracted and cultivated in a lab. Next, CRISPR technology alters the DNA by activating the fetal hemoglobin gene. Finally, these modified stem cells are reintroduced into the patient's body with a working version of the fetal hemoglobin gene. These altered cells have the potential to support the generation of healthy red blood cells that have proven effective in affected patients.

LOOKING AHEAD

CRISPR has transformed from a bacterial defense mechanism discovered a few decades ago into a genetic and medical breakthrough. Its ability to accurately correct DNA sequences can provide new strategies for treating once unapproachable diseases, such as Huntington's disease and sickle cell anemia. Thus, CRISPR alters our view of biology and changes notions about the boundaries of the possible in health and technology.

The journey of CRISPR is far from over. It is a story of discovery, promise, and the challenges of wielding the power to rewrite the blueprint of life itself. In Chapter 7, I will explore how this groundbreaking tool can be harnessed to address anxiety, offering new hope for treatment.

6

Gene Therapy & The Ethical Frontier

Enhancing Minds or Crossing Lines?

EVENTS CAN CHANGE the trajectory of disease, for good or ill.

Despite my uneven childhood and adolescence, I felt my anxiety was manageable throughout my early twenties as an undergraduate student. One of the most important decisions I made in my life was summer employment at Glacier National Park (GNP) in Montana, granting me a new sense of freedom.

That began a long love affair with GNP and Mother Nature. Mountaineering became my passion, and I often found myself in precarious situations, such as a daring off-trail hike by myself (note to reader: dumb idea!): Ptarmigan tunnel to Ahern pass via the Pinnacle Wall goat trail. This route was beautifully described by the climbing icon of GNP Gordon Edwards in his book A Climber's Guide to Glacier National Park (published in 1995 by Glacier Natural History Association, in cooperation with Falcon Press Publishing Co., Inc., Helena, Montana.)

Here is Edward's first sentence in describing this route: "Distance along goat trail about four miles. Class 2 and 3 most of the way, but a slip off the trail would be fatal in many places. ... Follow the excellent goat trail westward on that ridge, up to the bottom of the HUGE cliff, and then around onto the great scree slope on the north face. (Shun the goat trail that goes onto the north side of the ridge earlier, for it ends in awful cliffs.)"

Did I take his advice?

Being in my early twenties and not having a fully developed frontal lobe, I followed the goat trail to the north side and soon found myself on a ten-inch ledge, pinned like a pancake on the face of a 3,000-foot cliff! At that moment, I realized I had made the ultimate rookie mountaineering mistake: trusting a goat's sense of direction. Goats may look confident on cliffs, but they are not filling out liability waivers.

I was shaken with fear. I knew I had to calm down, so I took a minute to collect myself. I realized that to solve this problem, I would have to step off the ledge and go downward until I could find a foothold. I secured a foothold, and by lowering my head level, I could get around the ledge wall impasse and make it to safety.

My other impactful mountaineering experience was encountering a grizzly sow and her two cubs at less than 25 yards. I escaped injury, but the event still produces nightmares 30 years later.

These two specific events served as additional triggers for an anxiety diagnosis later on in my life. Here is why: Facing a frightening situation that triggers a fight-or-flight response and potentially results in a lasting psychological impact. In some cases, it can even lead to long-term psychological effects like post-traumatic stress or anxiety.

Both situations triggered fear and a sense of powerlessness, along with a perceived danger of death, all traits of distressing events that can leave lasting effects. These experiences can result in increased anxiety levels and heightened vigilance over time, potentially leading to the onset of an anxiety disorder.

Yet, despite facing some terrifying situations, GNP has had an enduring, positive impact on me. Amidst the wilderness and the uncertainty, I discovered friendship and stability through my relationships with co-workers and, most of all, through meeting my future wife. Twenty-five-plus years later, she has stood by and supported this knucklehead, for which I am entirely grateful.

NATURE, NURTURE & THE USE OF GENE THERAPY

Chronic anxiety has emerged as a significant global health concern, often described as an epidemic due to its widespread prevalence and the substantial burden it places on individuals and healthcare systems. Recent studies indicate that a considerable portion of patients suffering from anxiety remain untreated, with estimates suggesting that around 60 percent of individuals do not receive any form of intervention for their anxiety disorders (Fattouh et al., 2019).

Moreover, a significant subset of patients exhibit resistance to available treatments, with reports indicating that approximately 22 percent of individuals with anxiety disorders do not respond adequately to conventional therapeutic approaches (Figure 6.1). These findings underscore the importance of developing novel therapeutic options to address anxiety effectively within the general population.

Figure 6.1: The Overall Health Outcomes for Patients Diagnosed With an Anxiety Disorder

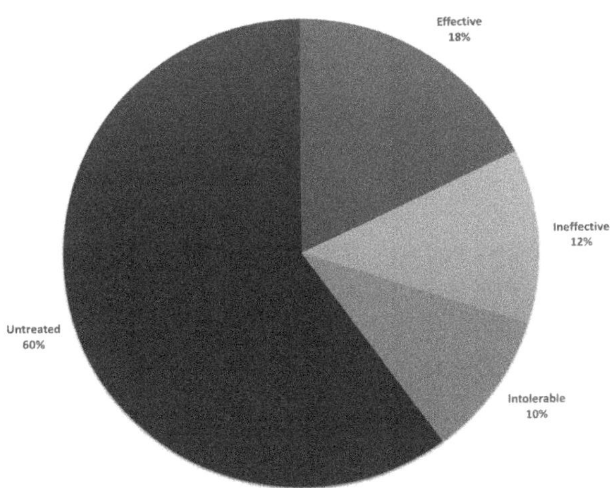

Note: A high proportion of the 60 percent did not receive any treatment, highlighting an issue in access to and provision of care. Of those who underwent treatment, 18 percent found it successful, 12 percent deemed it ineffective, and 10 percent encountered side effects.

Clearly, innovative approaches are urgently needed to address the unmet need for effective treatments for chronic anxiety.

My experiences at GNP provide a good example of how nature and nurture interact to create disease. However, what if we could change the "nature" part, the biological pathways? Gene therapy is currently being developed as a potential treatment for various diseases and conditions, and thus, the boundaries of what is considered possible in science are being pushed.

However, this new capability to enhance or modify also creates ethical issues.

To the point: Is it right to interfere with the genes that determine our psyche? Editing genes is like Photoshop: one wrong click and your ethical considerations suddenly go viral. In this chapter, we will explore how gene therapy is on the verge of becoming an innovative technique that can bring a revolution in the field of medicine while at the same time posing some ethical concerns concerning the alteration of human beings.

ETHICAL CONSIDERATIONS

Genetic techniques raise dilemmas regarding the lasting impacts of gene engineering. The capacity to alter brain circuits via gene therapy might pose untoward effects, such as alterations in abilities or character traits. The possibility of unequal accessibility due to the costs of these cutting-edge treatments is also a real concern.

Access

As is the case with any new technology, the new therapeutics will undoubtedly carry a high price tag. For example, according to the American Academy of Family Physicians, the list price of Casgevy, the first approved CRISPR-based gene editing therapy for sickle cell disease and transfusion-dependent beta-thalassemia (TDT), is approximately $2.2 million *per patient*!

The potential for social inequality, if only the wealthy can afford these advancements, underscores the need for equitable access to this technology. It also highlights the importance of strong oversight and well-defined ethical principles to ensure that these advancements positively impact patients mindfully and fairly.

Potential Health Disparities

Access and fairness are also factors to consider in gene therapies due to their high costs and the need for specialized infrastructure for administration and monitoring services. The concern is that these treatments are exclusive to a privileged few individuals. How can we ensure gene therapy breakthroughs reach those who need them most without worsening health disparities?

Safety

The ability to change brain chemistry through gene therapy also poses safety concerns. Any action that alters brain pathways may lead to unforeseen, long-lasting outcomes, such as off-target effects or irreversible changes in cognitive and emotional capabilities. This is particularly true of CRISPR/Cas9 therapeutics, which directly modify the actual genome through DNA modifications.

CRISPR

Off-target modifications might have profound implications within the neurons, perhaps interfering with crucial genes associated with brain operations and potentially causing cognitive or neurological challenges. Editing the DNA of neurons, particularly in humans, raises ethical issues about the unintended changes to neural networks that underlie certain behaviors. Using CRISPR to calm neurons is like hitting the mute button at a family holiday dinner: effective but morally complex.

Unlike most cells in the body with reproductive capabilities, neurons lack this capacity; therefore, any adjustments are expected to endure permanently. The lasting impacts of changing DNA to address conditions such as anxiety or Alzheimer's remain unclear. However, any changes induced by the application of CRISPR would *not* carry over to future offspring. This is because DNA modifications in the parent do not carry over into reproductive cells, including sperm and eggs.

RNAi

Another gene therapy technique I will discuss in the coming chapters is RNA interference (**RNAi**). RNAi is a biological process in which small RNA molecules, such as short hairpin RNA (**shRNA)**, silence specific genes by degrading their messenger RNA (mRNA), thereby preventing protein production. Unlike CRISPR, which permanently alters the DNA, RNAi provides a reversible and temporary approach, allowing precise regulation of gene expression *without* modifying the genetic code. This makes RNAi a potentially safer and more adaptable option for addressing conditions like anxiety.

Because an RNAi therapeutic can result in **gene silencing** without permanently altering the DNA, ethical concerns regarding changes in anxiety or improved memory may make it more acceptable. The downside of RNAi is that because it does not produce a permanent change, the effects are shorter-lived and, therefore, may require repeated treatments to sustain any clinical benefit. Our data and other studies suggest that a single RNAi treatment would last anywhere from several weeks to six months based on preclinical model data (Kim et al., 2023; Pasi et al., 2017).

While my own company's research on rodents has displayed encouraging outcomes, transferring this to human use demands meticulous assessment. Clinical trials are needed to guarantee that these therapies do not create hazards beyond their intended use.

NEUROENHANCEMENT

So far, we've looked at ethics in the treatment of disease. Another potential ethical quagmire is whether these therapies could enhance cognition in normal, healthy individuals. The noticeable memory enhancements resulting from *HTR2A* gene regulation in *normal* rodents (to be discussed in the coming chapters) raise the prospect of utilizing these treatments to address neuropsychiatric conditions as well as boost regular cognitive abilities. This particular scenario leads us to the realm of neuroenhancement. For instance, should we permit actions intended to elevate the capabilities of healthy individuals beyond a standard level? If so, how should we oversee and manage the societal repercussions of potentially creating cognitive benefits for a privileged few?

This new technology can be employed beyond treating neuropsychiatric conditions to enhance our mental abilities over time as part of a comprehensive plan for overall well-being and graceful aging (Figure 6.2). The basic idea is to alter gene expression to improve cognitive skills in individuals who are already healthy. As stated above, this could result in ethical concerns that such enhancement could widen the gap between different societal groups, as only select populations would have the means to benefit from these cutting-edge treatments.

Additionally, blurring the distinction between treating a condition and improving natural cognitive skills could raise concerns about fairness, consent, and societal consequences.

Figure 6.2: Applications of Gene Therapy: From Cognitive Deficits to Enhancing Abilities in Healthy Individuals

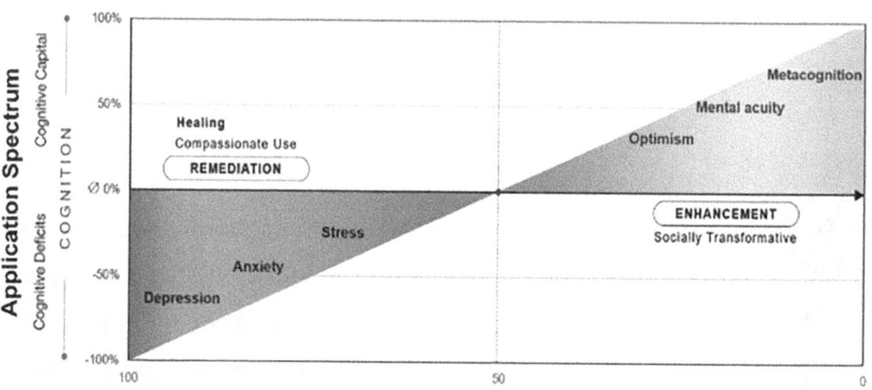

Note: On the left, therapies are used to manage conditions like depression, anxiety, and stress, falling under "compassionate use" for healing. Moving along the spectrum, the focus shifts to improving functions such as hopefulness and mental sharpness, which could impact society by enhancing cognitive reserve. The spectrum showcases both methods for therapy and potential advancements for cognitive enhancement.

As technology progresses, these ethical dilemmas surrounding longevity and cognitive enhancement will likely become more evident. Questions emerge about the availability of these life-prolongation technologies and how they will be incorporated into society.

Additionally, there is a risk of outcomes such as enhancing cognitive well-being in a manner that interferes with natural aging processes and potentially worsening age-related inequalities in health and wealth. These matters necessitate thoughtful, ethical deliberation to guarantee that such improvements in cognitive health contribute to the well-being of all members of society equitably and responsibly. As we move closer to applying these advancements, it is crucial to maintain an ongoing dialogue on ethics that involves researchers, healthcare providers, ethicists, and the general public. Our top priority should be maintaining a balance between pushing the boundaries of science to address issues like anxiety and cognitive decline and upholding safety and fairness. Ethical considerations regarding the proper use of these powerful technologies are paramount for any start-up company using gene therapy.

The future development of gene therapy for cognitive enhancement will also significantly depend on public opinion and policy decisions rather than scientific progress alone. While scientific progress may pave the way for technologies, ultimately, the societal consensus will decide the extent to which these advancements are integrated into our daily lives.

The ethical considerations related to cognitive enhancement are thorny indeed. The aim of enhancing qualities such as memory or intelligence, rather than curing diseases, forces society to rethink its beliefs about fairness, self-identity, and equality.

Public opinion can significantly influence the acceptance or rejection of such treatments. The public's perception of enhancement could lead to its widespread acceptance or rejection. Cognitive enhancement methods might be welcomed if perceived to enhance health and promote fairness. However, they could face opposition if viewed as creating an unfair playing field that could intensify social disparities while disrupting humanity's fundamental nature (Table 6.1).

Table 6.1: Comparison of Ethical Considerations & Societal Impacts of Therapeutic vs. Enhancement-Focused Uses of Gene Therapy

CATEGORY	EXAMPLES	ETHICAL CONSIDERATIONS	SOCIETAL IMPACT
Therapeutic Use	Treating anxiety, depression, Alzheimer's disease	Focused on alleviating illness and improving quality of life; risks are often weighed against the severity of the condition	Positive impact on healthcare outcomes and mental health; can reduce the burden of disease
Enhancement Use	Improving memory, enhancing focus, reducing normal stress	Raises concerns about fairness, consent and human identity; may increase societal inequality if accessibility is limited	Potential for societal division based on access to enhancements; could alter perceptions of "normal" human ability

Universally accepted policies will also help oversee the balance between fostering innovation and guarding against potential misuse of such technology. Governments and regulatory bodies, for example, must strike a balance between promoting innovation and protecting against misuse or unintended consequences. The intertwining of opinion and policy is evident here, and our collective perception and support or lack of support of these advancements will influence the governmental regulatory frameworks that define their trajectory.

In summary, the possibility of using gene therapy to enhance cognition extends beyond technological advancements to societal realms. Our discussions, regulations, and moral limits will dictate whether this innovation is utilized for healing or potential misuse. Navigating this ethical terrain carefully is essential for making responsible decisions.

7

Targeting & Rewiring Anxiety

The 5-HT2A Receptor & CRISPR-Cas9

OUR CHOICES CAN also affect health outcomes.

While anxiety was becoming a constant, it didn't define me or my life. Things got so bad at home in my senior year of high school that I considered leaving, not out of the usual teenage defiance, but as a matter of survival.

Staying with one of my best friends seemed like a safe bet. I spent so much time at his house anyway, and his parents knew all about my family situation. They did not just tolerate me hanging around; they were genuinely kind (a foreign concept to me then). I would sit at their dinner table, watching in mild fascination as they communicated like actual humans; they were supportive, engaged, and civil, resembling a documentary on how families are supposed to work.

However, even at the advanced age of 17, I knew that running from a mess into someone else's tidy living room was an escape hatch, not a long-term solution. Plus, let us face it: no matter how much my friend's family might like me, no one signs up to foster a surly, academically driven teenager indefinitely.

My older sister had successfully navigated her way out of our family chaos and was enrolled in college, proving there was a way out.

So, following her inspiring example, I completed my college applications, took the SAT, and secured early admission to UC Davis.

Seemingly, my mother shared the sentiment. Upon graduating from high school, I received an interesting gift: a brand new suitcase! Trust me, I made great use of it. A few weeks after my high school graduation ceremony, I boldly gathered my stuff and bid farewell to my hometown, successfully executing my escape plan and embarking on my academic journey.

During my adolescence, I felt like I was in constant survival mode. Leaving for college was not just about academics; it was also my chance to escape the turmoil and rewrite my future.

By that time, anxiety had already rewired my brain and left a lasting impact on how I dealt with stress, fear, and even hope for change. This is the difficulty of chronic anxiety: it is no longer a reaction to a specific cue; it becomes a part of a person at the biological level, influencing how the brain and body respond to the world.

However, what if we could rewire those responses, targeting the mechanisms that perpetuate anxiety at their source? In this chapter, I will explore how CRISPR technology addresses anxiety, specifically at the genetic level. This approach is not only a therapeutic strategy, but it holds the key to completely overhauling the brain's circuitry and giving those suffering from anxiety a new beginning.

MODULATING THE 5-HT2A RECEPTOR

The COVID-19 pandemic was a time of uncertainty and fear when the world had to deal with new challenges to our resilience, challenges that most of us had not experienced in our lifetimes. It was a period of social distancing, uncertainty, and an increased sense of frailty. The data regarding the impact the COVID-19 pandemic has had on the number of anxiety and depression cases is alarming. Both disorders have increased by a factor of four in both women and men (Figure 7.1).

Figure 7.1: Global Prevalence of Anxiety and Depression Before and During the COVID-19 Pandemic, Across Different Age Groups

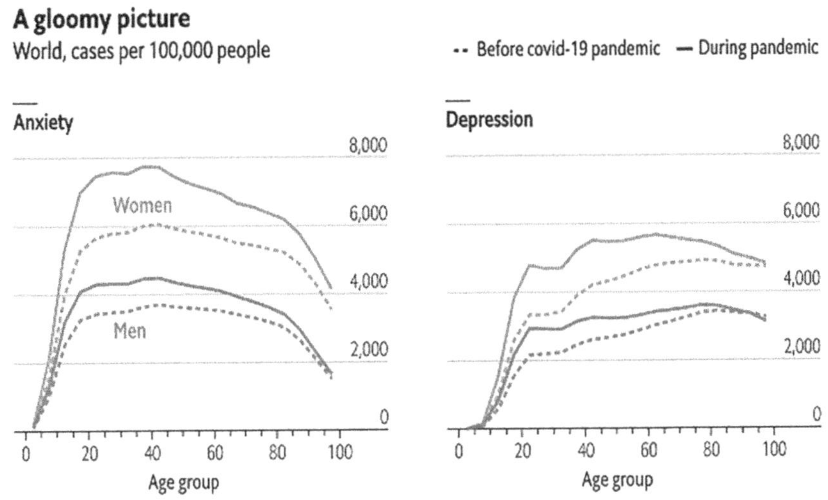

Note: Anxiety (left panel) and depression (right panel) show an increase in cases per 100,000 people during the pandemic (solid lines) compared to pre-pandemic levels (dashed lines). Women (blue lines) are more affected than men (red lines) in both disorders, particularly in younger age groups (Santomauro et al., 2021).

The pandemic also increased the challenges of anxiety on a global level and, at the same time, highlighted the demand for new approaches to dealing with mental health problems, approaches of the very kind I had been interested in for so long.

CRISPR, a technological advancement that was derived from a bacterial defense mechanism, has the potential to change the way that psychological disorders, such as anxiety, are managed.

As discussed in Chapter 2, the 5-HT2A receptor plays a key role in anxiety and depression, and traditional treatments with serotonin reuptake inhibitors (SSRIs) often have many side effects, offer limited effectiveness, and require daily use. This highlights the great need for a new generation of therapeutic options to address anxiety (as well as other neuropsychiatric disorders, including Alzheimer's, schizophrenia, and depression). I believe that gene therapy targeting specific receptors and neural pathways will usher in a new era of therapeutics, achieving greater efficacy and fewer side effects than current legacy treatments.

STARTING IN THE DISH

In designing therapeutics to treat human disease, a logistical flow of experiments must be completed before testing in humans. The first step usually involves **in vitro** experiments, which means "outside the body." These experiments usually involve neurons grown in small chambers.

The advantage of this approach is that you have a homogenous population of neurons (in other words, all the neurons are about the same), and the researcher can control all potential variables, isolating those they are testing. In addition, experiments using neurons in vitro may produce faster results as these experiments can be carried out in hours or days instead of weeks or months using **in vivo** (within the body) animal models. Finally, neurons in a culture are more accessible for visualization and manipulation. You can more easily apply techniques such as electrophysiology, cell imaging, or gene editing (e.g., CRISPR).

Of course, the limitation of in vitro models is that they do not fully recapitulate the vast complexity of a living organism.

Therefore, the results may not translate into what occurs in vivo. Thus, it is only a starting point, and similar experiments should be confirmed in vivo to account for whole-brain interactions.

My own company's first set of experiments employed CRISPR/Cas9 to target the knockdown of the 5-HT2A receptor in vitro, using cultured neurons. In this section, I'll present some of our results.

TARGETING THE 5-HT2A GENE REDUCES EXCITABILITY

The following discussion summarizes findings from a recent peer-reviewed article published in *PNAS Nexus* (Rohn et al., 2023). The first step in this process was to design the proper **guide RNA (gRNA)** to ensure that only the *HTR2A* gene was targeted. As shown in Figure 7.2, we created a validated gRNA, one that appeared to be a good candidate for testing in vitro using mouse cortical neurons.

Figure 7.2: Using a CRISPR/Cas9 Gene-Editing Tool to Deactivate the HTR2A Gene

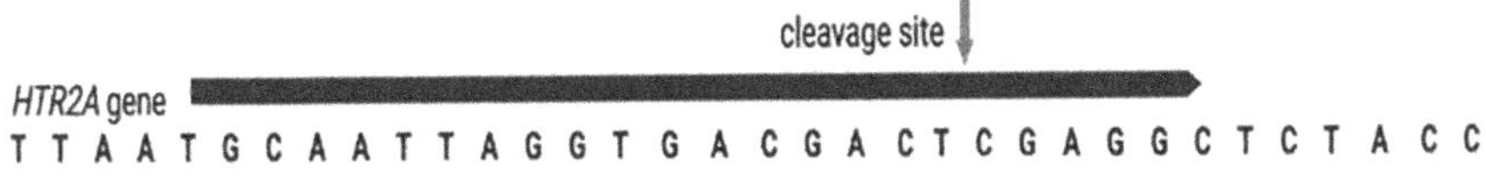

- No predicted off-target sites
- Frameshift frequency 88.6%

Note: The HTR2A gene is found on mouse chromosome 14, producing one particular type of protein: the 5-HT2A receptor. The black line represents the guide RNA (gRNA) and tells the Cas9 enzyme where to cut the DNA. The Cas9 enzyme will cut the DNA between two specific letters, T and C, which are part of the genetic code (represented by the arrow). This gRNA is predicted to be very specific, meaning it is not expected to accidentally cut other parts of the DNA (off-target sites). After the cut, there is an 88.6 percent chance that repairing this cut causes a frameshift and introduces a premature stop codon and non-functional protein (see Chapter 5 for more detail on this protein production). A color version of this image can be viewed at getfitnow.com/extras.

An essential tenet of research is that it is **hypothesis-driven.** In this experiment, our working hypothesis was based on the known excitatory properties of the 5-HT2A receptor. We hypothesized that decreasing the expression of this receptor in the neurons would lead to a *decrease* in the electrical activity of neurons in culture. Our hypothesis was supported by the data, which indicated a significant reduction in neuronal electrical activity following treatment with CRISPR/Cas9 (Figure 7.3). In essence, we told the 5-HT2A receptor to take a permanent coffee break, and the neurons responded by dialing down their activity. (Like cutting the cable on a noisy neighbor's television, we finally got some peace and quiet in the network.) This validation was a critical step for our next series of in vivo experiments.

Figure 7.3: Using CRISPR/Cas9 Technology to Target and Disrupt the HTR2A Gene in Mouse Brain Neurons

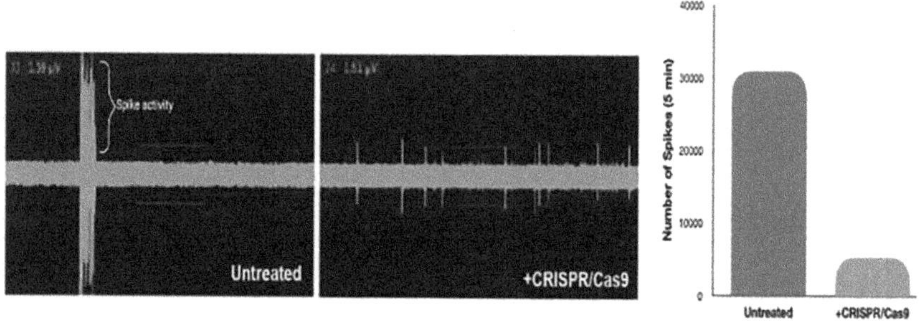

Note: The left panel (Untreated) displays the electrical spikes recorded from untreated neurons, showing strong spike activity. The right panel (+CRISPR/Cas9) shows that neurons treated with CRISPR/Cas9 to deactivate the HTR2A gene had much less electrical activity. The graph on the right quantifies this effect, revealing a significant drop in spikes (electrical signals) after the treatment (green bar), suggesting that knocking out this gene affects neuron firing.

TARGETING THE 5-HT2A GENE DECREASES ANXIETY

The next big question was whether downregulating the 5-HT2A receptor would impact anxiety. These preliminary results marked an essential proof of concept, namely, that gene therapy can be a viable therapeutic strategy. However, seeing an impact on neurons cultured in a laboratory setting is one thing. It is a whole other matter to see any effect on the behavior of a living organism. To test this, we turned to rodent models, starting with wild-type (normal, disorder-free) mice.

Using CRISPR to tweak genes and tackle anxiety is not exactly a fast-food solution. We don't expect to see results instantly. It is more like preparing a stew on low heat: the therapy must reach the right brain cells, cut the correct gene, and then wait for the body to remove the old proteins and bring about the desired changes.

This process took about five weeks in mice, which is pretty quick in scientific terms, but still enough for the mice to wonder why they were suddenly glowing green under UV light (thanks to the fluorescent marker we added to track the therapy). After ensuring that our genetic editing tool targeted the right part of the brain (the anxiety circuits), we found out that our CRISPR therapy worked as expected. It achieved its target of editing a specific gene (*HTR2A*), which is linked with anxiety.

So, what happened to the behavior of the mice? Less of the 5-HT2A receptor proteins, less stress signaling, and perhaps fewer "mouse panic attacks" were observed. However, this is not all; the mice also changed their overall behavior.

The first big test we conducted was the so-called marble burying test, a model of stress in mice. The more marbles the mouse hides, the more anxious it is. When the mice received our gene therapy, they buried significantly fewer marbles, meaning they were less anxious (perhaps a mouse version of Marie Kondo).

This was the first time that gene therapy had been shown to alter anxiety, and believe me, the entire group at our company reacted with expletives. The revised version: "These results are ****ing incredible!" Yes, CRISPR chilled out the mice, and yes, this represents a great hope for treating anxiety in the future.

To put these results in perspective, we also compared our results to diazepam (Valium), the gold-standard medication for lowering anxiety. It is essential to point out a fundamental difference in this comparative experiment: the effects of Valium were assessed *acutely* within 30 minutes after dosing. In contrast, CRISPR/Cas9-treated mice were not evaluated for anxiety until five weeks later. Using this comparative strategy, we found that CRISPR/Cas9 treatment ultimately led to a comparable decrease in anxiety as diazepam (Figure 7.4).

Figure 7.4: Comparison of the Anti-Anxiety Effects of Gene-Editing Therapy (CRISPR/Cas9) and the Standard Anti-Anxiety Medication Diazepam (Valium)

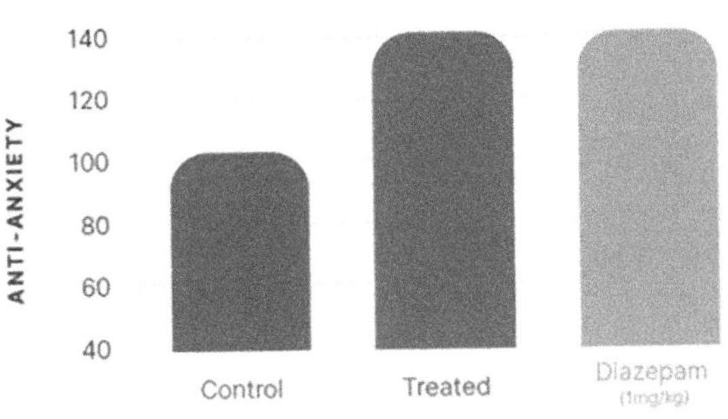

Summary: We devised a sophisticated way of delivering gene therapy, which carried CRISPR/Cas9 and a genetic map (guide RNA) to target and turn off 5-HT2A receptors in particular regions of the brain associated with anxiety.

Simplified: We developed a way to eliminate those neurons that tend to overact.

Translation: We found a way to snip out the bits of the brain that generate anxious behavior.

After running three different mouse stress tests, including the aforementioned marble-burying, we saw a reduction in anxiety-related behaviors.

IMPLICATIONS FOR ANXIETY TREATMENT

What does this mean? Not only did we show that CRISPR can calm anxious mice, but we also proved it might be possible to permanently tweak specific traits (like the stress response) in the long term. This could be a game-changer for developing next-generation psychiatric medications, involving less trial-and-error and more targeted solutions. Imagine a one-and-done fix for chronic anxiety, no daily pills required. It is still early days, but the mice seem to approve!

When we consider the possibilities of CRISPR technology beyond addressing anxiety issues alone, these results also signal a new chapter in medicine. We envision a scenario where therapies go beyond alleviating the outward symptoms of mental health conditions and tackle their fundamental origins. In place of relying on daily doses of medication, gene editing presents the potential for enduring solutions, even requiring just a single intervention to fundamentally recalibrate the brain's biochemical processes for lasting benefits. By tweaking specific genes that influence mood or behavior, scientists could help balance brain chemistry in ways that current medications cannot.

IMPLICATIONS FOR OTHER DISORDERS

Apart from anxiety disorders, CRISPR also shows potential for addressing other mental health conditions such as depression, ADHD, and schizophrenia. By adjusting the expression of specific genes that impact emotions and actions, gene therapy interventions could restore the balance of brain chemistry in a manner that existing drugs cannot achieve.

It may seem like a plotline out of a science fiction story; however, trials for treatments based on CRISPR are currently in progress for various ailments like sickle cell anemia (discussed earlier in this book) and specific cancer types, as researchers strive to improve the technology further. It will not be long before its usage extends to other health issues (Table 7.1). The goal is to transition gene therapy from the confines of the lab to clinical applications within the next ten years, paving the way for these transformative treatments to reach more individuals.

Table 7.1: Mental Health Disorders, Their Related Target Genes/Receptors & Potential Outcomes of Using Gene Therapy

MENTAL HEALTH DISORDER	TARGET GENES/RECEPTORS	POTENTIAL OUTCOME
Anxiety	5-HT2A Receptor	Reduced anxiety
Depression	Serotonin Transporter (SERT)	Improved mood
PTSD	Glucocorticoid Receptor (GR)	Reduction in stress response
Schizophrenia	Dopamine Receptor (DRD2)	Reduction in psychotic symptoms
ADHD	Dopamine Transporter (DAT1)	Improved attention and focus

The adventure is only beginning, and scenarios of CRISPR altering the narrative of health care and changing the lives of many individuals who face anxiety and other conditions are unfolding. It is a future filled with hope and optimism—and we are on the cusp of making it a reality.

8

RNA Therapeutics

Silencing the 5-HT2A Receptor to Tame Anxiety

THE PERILOUS ADVENTURE of graduate school felt like a slow-motion train wreck, minus the excitement.

My social skills could have been best described as "nonexistent." Pair that with my top-notch graduate program, complete with egos so large they could barely fit through the lab doors, and the competitive atmosphere (think "The Hunger Games," except with more pipettes and fewer explosions). As half of my graduate class fell by the wayside, I had never felt more alone. Much of it was a self-imposed isolation; I had surrounded myself with impenetrable protective walls.

At some point, I had a eureka moment, probably around when I was eating ramen for the third meal in a row. No, I did not finally understand electrophysiology—I am still fuzzy on that one—but I did realize I needed help. Seeking counseling services was my first brilliant decision during those years. Through a much-needed reality check, I started to understand that perhaps being cold, distant, and mildly terrifying to everyone around me was not the best strategy for long-term success, personal or professional.

Lest anyone think this is a sob story, let me assure you I was never clinically depressed, nor did I entertain any "why me?" sentiments. I did not wallow in self-pity. If anything, anxiety had an odd way of fueling my determination. I was a lonely, emotionally distant, semi-dysfunctional mess, but I had goals that kept me marching forward, even if I did not exactly know where I was going. Nevertheless, in the end, the journey—however isolating and frustrating—revealed the resilience I never knew I had. Frankly, that resilience is the only reason I survived to write about it.

Upon reflection, many of these behaviors, including isolation, focus, and emotional detachment, were, in fact, manifestations of anxiety. The barriers I erected and my fixation on work were coping mechanisms to manage an overwhelming fear of failure and judgment. These behaviors of isolating, fixating on work, and avoiding people were manifestations of anxiety.

It was not just psychological; it was *biological.* Anxiety had become a part of me and had altered my thought process and my perception of the world. I sought counseling during that period, and it helped me to recognize the causes of my problems, but it also raised more questions: Could anxiety be treated at its core? Could the very bodily mechanisms that define these behaviors be rewritten?

RNA THERAPY

The impressive results of CRISPR that we obtained by targeting the *HTR2A* gene demonstrate the great promise of gene editing tools. What about treating non-lethal disorders such as anxiety, depression, and memory impairments that affect millions of people worldwide, and for which CRISPR technology may not be an attractive approach? An alternative approach is using RNA therapy.

RNA therapy involves utilizing RNA molecules, like messenger RNA (**mRNA**) and small interfering RNA (**siRNA** or **shRNA**). These treatments can reduce the presence of a malformed protein by using siRNA or shRNA to break down the mRNA responsible for regulating gene expression. Acting on RNA means acting one step below the DNA. The rationale is that mRNA is made and destroyed all the time, so regulating this part of gene expression should be a safer approach compared to changing the DNA by using CRISPR. Think of it this way: RNA therapy addresses the problem at the "Post-It™ note stage" rather than rewriting the entire definitive instruction manual. It is a bit like intercepting a grocery list *before* someone buys 50 pounds of kale: they might not even notice the change, but everyone is happier in the end.

Imagine your mind as a symphony where each gene acts as a unique musician, shaping your emotional harmony and balance. When specific musicians play off-key and disrupt the harmony, this may lead to anxiety or other mental issues. This is where shRNA and siRNA step in, like conductors who can selectively silence or calm down the instruments (or genes) responsible for the disharmony. Simply put, after interrupting the mRNA, shRNA, and siRNA work to quiet overly active or troublesome genes. This transient hushing aids in reinstating equilibrium. By calming specific genes, these RNA molecules represent a method to adjust the brain's symphony and enhance mental serenity, delicately silencing the molecular chatter that throws everything out of harmony.

In contrast to CRISPR gene therapy, which focuses on making lasting changes, RNA therapy offers an adaptable approach that can be adjusted over time to achieve the desired therapeutic outcomes. This flexibility is an attractive alternative to CRISPR in neuropsychiatric disorders where precise management of receptor levels might be necessary.

KNOCKING DOWN THE 5-HT2A RECEPTOR IN VITRO

To evaluate the potential effectiveness of RNA therapy, my team developed a shRNA designed to target the 5-HT2A receptor mRNA.

In contrast to our CRISPR therapeutic, which we named Cog-101, this RNA therapeutic was designated as Cog-201. Many of the summarized results presented here have been published in full in the peer-reviewed journals *Translational Psychiatry* and *Genomic Psychiatry* (Rohn et al., 2024a; Rohn et al., 2024b).

We followed a similar experimental design to our CRISPR approach (see Chapter 7). To ensure that Cog-201 was effective, we also incorporated a green fluorescent protein as a marker to ensure that the targeting was specific to the brain, like pasting a small neon sign on the neurons that said, "Cog-201 has struck here."

How does shRNA work? shRNA functions by creating a "self-destruct" signal for the instructions of a specific protein. When introduced into a cell, shRNA folds into a double-stranded structure that complements the mRNA of the target protein.

Cells naturally recognize double-stranded mRNA as a signal for destruction, which activates a defense mechanism. A protein complex known as RISC (RNA-induced silencing complex) then degrades the targeted mRNA, preventing it from being translated into a protein. Without its mRNA instructions, the cell can no longer produce the protein, resulting in its downregulation. In simple terms, if mRNA is a recipe for making a protein, double-stranded mRNA is a red flag that tells the cell to throw the recipe away before it's used.

The main component of shRNA Cog-201 is designed to eliminate the 5-HT2A receptor mRNA, akin to cutting the power line to a stress signal. We even included a "scrambled" version as a control—a kind of genetic placebo without any functionality—to confirm that our real tool was not acting by chance. The results? Cog-201 reduced the mRNA levels of its target, 5-HT2A, inhibiting the overactive neurons. (Imagine neurons going from a fireworks show to a low-key candlelight dinner). We also used some electrical tests to determine the number of neuron spikes, which helped us understand that Cog-201 was actually suppressing *brain activity* to some extent. This was in line with what we had observed when we used CRISPR in our earlier experiments.

However, the real work in science continues beyond the lab bench. We then tested Cog-201 on live mice to determine if such suppression of neuronal activity changes anxiety-like behavior. Using the standard **light/dark choice test**—a mouse's version of "Do I dare leave my comfort zone?"—we found that Cog-201-treated mice were far braver than their untreated counterparts. They preferred to explore the brightly lit areas and spent more time in those regions, thus indicating that they had reduced anxiety levels (Figure 8.1).

Figure 8.1: The Impact of Two Treatments on Mice's Anxiety Levels

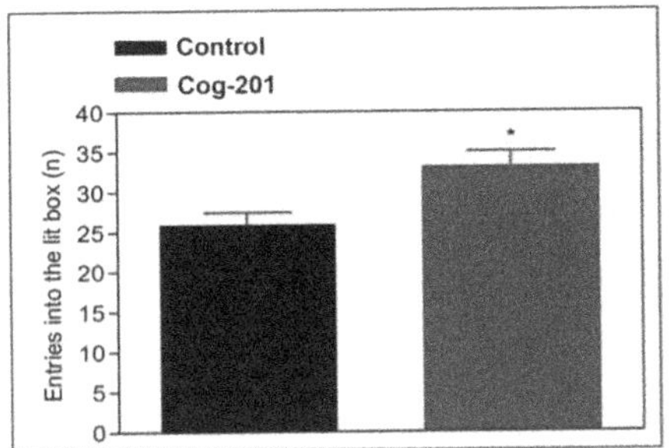

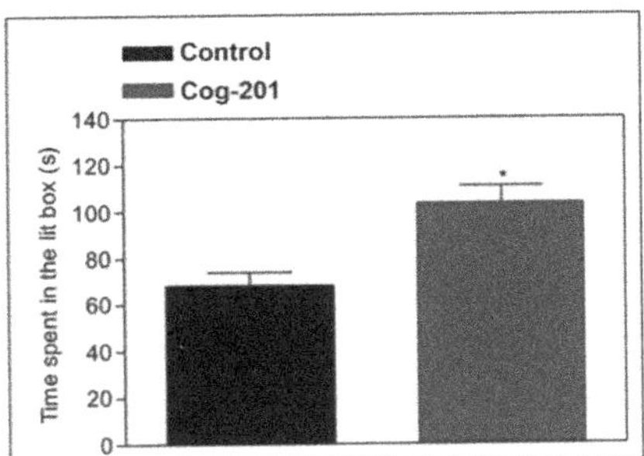

Note: Data from a light-dark box method test, where the black bars indicate mice that did not receive treatment (control), and the blue bars depict mice that received Cog-201. The graph on the left shows how frequently the mice went into the illuminated box area.

Observably, mice that underwent RNA therapy displayed a greater frequency of entering the lit box than the control group. On the right, the graph shows how long mice stayed in box areas; mice that underwent

Cog-201 therapy lingered noticeably longer in the lit box, which suggests lower anxiety levels were observed among them.

Analysis confirms these differences are statistically significant.

So, what is the takeaway? Cog-201 is shaping up to be a strong candidate for turning nervous mice (and maybe someday, anxious humans) into more relaxed versions of themselves. It is another win for science and mice who have had enough of living in the dark.

KNOCKING DOWN THE 5-HT2A RECEPTOR IMPROVES MEMORY

In a nice reversal of expectations, we also discovered that not only does Cog-201 take the edge off anxiety, but it also enhances memory! While the scientific community has been split on whether manipulating the 5-HT2A receptor enhances or hinders memory, studies have shown mixed results. The variations in the outcomes of these studies may arise from factors such as the brain mechanisms overseeing different memory types or the drug dosage. Also, some drugs might influence other brain regions apart from memory-related ones.

Research conducted with medications that inhibit the 5-HT2A has yielded varying outcomes. Some medications enhance memory function, while others do not demonstrate this effect (Zhang & Stackman, 2015). In contrast, studies involving the reduction of receptor levels in rodents have indicated improved memory performance (Cohen, 2005). In human trials, the 5-HT2A receptor antagonist Mianserin, administered at a daily dosage of 15 mg, has been used to enhance memory retention and cognitive function (Poyurovsky et al., 2003).

Based on these varied findings, we wanted to know if the modulation of this receptor could enhance memory using Cog-201. To do this, we had to resort to the **novel object preference test**, a complicated way of saying, "Do rats get bored with the same things?" This is how it works:

First, the rats are placed in an open space, and the experimenter does not put any objects in the field (so the rats learn that the area is safe). Second, two identical objects are provided, and the rats are allowed to investigate. Third, the subject is presented with one object similar to the previous one, but the other is new and shiny, and the subject's preference is observed. If the rats go for the new object, it means their memory is on point—they remember the old one.

The results? It is safe to say that the lab floors trembled as our results shocked everyone. The Cog-201-treated rats were much more interested in the new object and spent 72 percent more time exploring it than non-treated rats (Figure 8.2). In rat terms, that is like acing a pop quiz after a power nap. The graphs also confirmed what we already knew: Cog-201 had a significant impact on memory and recognition.

So, not only does Cog-201 assist mice in relaxing, but it also appears to make rats little memory geniuses. If this continues, then we might need to rebrand it as an "all-in-one" gene therapy for anxiety and memory problems.

Figure 8.2: The Performance of Two Groups of Rats, One Treated With Cog-201 and One Left Untreated

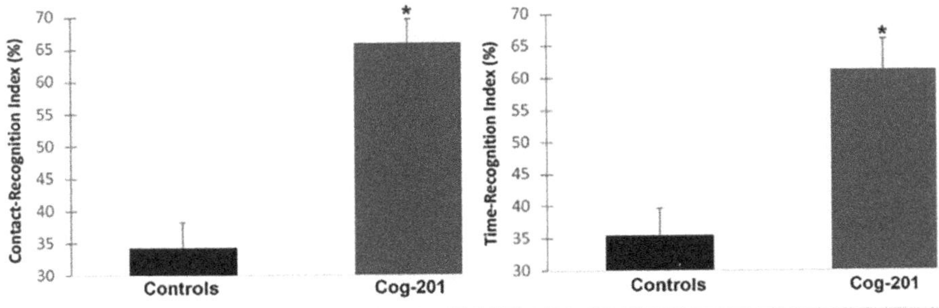

Note: One group was given gene therapy (represented by blue bars), and the other served as a control group (depicted by black bars). It illustrates their

performance in a memory assessment called the object recognition test. The graph on the left shows that the rats treated with gene therapy displayed significantly higher contact recognition index values than the control group represented by the black bars. This indicates that the rats treated with gene therapy tended to recognize and engage with the novel object more frequently than those in the control group. Treated rats also spent more time identifying the novel object than the control group, as indicated by the time recognition index in the right graph. These findings imply that Cog-201 enhanced memory and recognition in the treated rats.

These findings were another "eureka" moment: not only did we have a potential therapeutic benefit on anxiety, but the improved memory could help millions of people who struggle with Alzheimer's disease, for which current medications are hardly effective. Therefore, precisely targeting the HTR2A gene presents a novel therapeutic approach for treating chronic anxiety and age-related cognitive decline.

At this point, our team felt it was essential to put these findings in context with conventional medications used to treat anxiety and memory impairments. We compared Cog-101 and Cog-201 with diazepam (Valium, the gold standard for reducing anxiety) and donepezil (Aricept), the most popular medication for patients who exhibit dementia. Notably, the effects of diazepam and donepezil were assessed *acutely*, in contrast to Cog-101 or Cog-201, which were assessed up to five weeks after treatment. The results show that Cog-101 and -201 perform comparably to diazepam Valium and outperformed donepezil (Figure 8.3).

Figure 8.3: Treatment Effects Of Medication Vs. Cog-101 or Cog-201

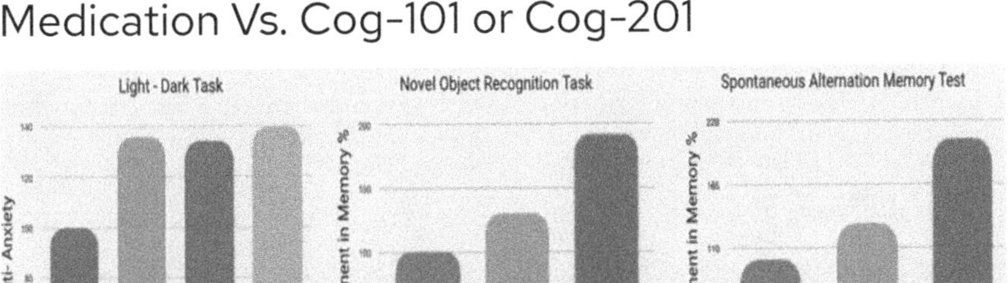

HOW RNA THERAPY WORKS TO TURN DOWN SEROTONIN "NOISE"

Picture your mind as a workplace brimming with employees (neurons) engaging in conversations to accomplish tasks. Their method of communication involves an abundance of telephones (**receptors**) and messages (**neurotransmitters**) zipping back and forth. Within this workplace, a phone line (the 5-HT2A receptor) tends to become overwhelmed when this line is incessantly ringing with calls (that is, high receptor activity).

This clamor makes it challenging for employees to concentrate on their duties and maintain focus. It is akin to everyone talking loudly, simultaneously, resulting in a cacophony of noise. To address this challenge, envision somehow decreasing the call traffic on this phone line. This action mirrors the downregulation of the 5-HT2A receptor, which essentially diminishes the noise level by reducing the volume of calls (receptor activity). This, in turn, can improve clarity and memory while also decreasing anxiety, as our research has shown.

LOOKING AHEAD

The positive outcomes witnessed with Cog-201 in alleviating anxiety through RNA interference marks the start of a promising journey. This method holds the promise to go beyond anxiety treatment and could potentially pave the way for addressing various neuropsychiatric conditions effectively and comprehensively. RNA therapy stands out for its adaptability due to its capacity to selectively pinpoint and regulate the functioning of almost any gene associated with mental health issues.

Disorders such as depression, schizophrenia, and Alzheimer's disease often involve disrupted gene expression or flawed protein synthesis. By adjusting or refining genes through RNA-based treatments, one could potentially rebalance these disruptions, as evidenced in our research on anxiety disorders. This ability to customize and adapt RNA therapies for patients and conditions could lead to a groundbreaking era of personalized psychiatric medicine.

Although our exploration of Cog-201 is still in the preclinical stage—that is, we haven't begun testing on humans—the extensive possibilities of RNA-based treatments for mental health conditions are remarkable. The potential to quiet genes without making permanent changes to the genetic code presents a precise approach that could revolutionize the field of mental health treatment.

Part III

Breaking Barriers in Brain Health & Gene Therapy

9

Treating Anxiety

Navigating the Blood-Brain Barrier

Anxiety can begin early in life, but its effects usually continue later in life.

During my childhood, my mother, preoccupied with her own needs, rarely offered the comfort or security that children crave. My sister recalls my cries as a baby being met with cold indifference or even harsh reprimands. As I grew older, I learned to internalize those early responses, hiding my fears and emotions rather than seeking solace, which left me to grapple with feelings of vulnerability that would linger well into adulthood.

I'm grateful for a kindly ultimatum from my wife-to-be: If the relationship was going to work, I had to step outside my comfort zone and talk to people, even if small talk felt like climbing a mental Everest. Slowly, her support and strategic plan, including giving me a social agenda for the day ahead, became our best practice against the social anxiety that often made me want to hide away.

Trust also became a cornerstone of our relationship. She even had to put her life in my hands on one of the most challenging mountaineering expeditions on the precarious cliffs of Mt. Wilbur in Glacier National Park. I vividly remember thinking that if she could trust me to lead her through that terrifying route, I could trust her to help me deal with my anxiety.

The resilience that I have been developing with help from my wife and my sister has helped me regain a sense of control. Paradoxically, while anxiety has always been a challenging part of my life, it has also driven me to build the strength to open up and reach out to people.

Cumulative, escalating anxiety is like trying to climb a cliff with no rope. While I could turn to relationships for support, addressing the biological cause of anxiety requires tackling an entirely different barrier that is built into my brain.

BIOLOGICAL CHALLENGES

This leads us to the **blood-brain barrier (BBB)**, a mechanical system that protects the brain from toxins in the bloodstream. As much as it protects us, the BBB poses a big problem for scientists who want to transport therapeutic molecules to treat anxiety and other brain diseases. In this chapter, I will try to explain why the BBB is such an obstacle and how scientists are working on new ways to break through it in order to provide better treatments for anxiety.

The BBB is a natural defense mechanism that acts like a barricade, safeguarding the brain from harmful substances in the bloodstream and, unfortunately, preventing many beneficial compounds from getting through as well. A key challenge in treating anxiety lies in ensuring that medications can breach this protective barrier to access the essential neurotransmitter systems within the brain.

Smaller, soluble molecules such as SSRIs can easily cross the barrier; however, larger and more intricate molecules, like the ones utilized in RNA-based treatments, face obstacles in passing through. The BBB also limits the success of developing therapeutics for central nervous system (CNS) disorders. Unique challenges emerge at the preclinical stage, partly due to the complexity of the human brain and partly due to the limited ability to study drug candidates in the relevant tissue environment.

More importantly, the aspect of the BBB creates multiple issues in drug penetration. Therapeutic drugs that show early promise during drug development often fail to clear subsequent clinical trials successfully due to their inability to cross the BBB. Nature is not easily tricked, and it has been estimated that more than 98 percent of small-molecule drugs and nearly 100 percent of large-molecule drugs are precluded from drug delivery to the brain as a result of the BBB (Pardridge, 2005)! Many promising therapeutics litter the highway of success because they cannot gain access to the CNS. Our gene therapies, Cog-101 and Cog-201, are no exceptions.

THE PURPOSE OF THE BBB

The **central nervous system (CNS)** encompasses the brain and spinal cord. It is bathed in a unique solution called **cerebral spinal fluid (CSF)** that cushions and protects these vital organs against damage. This fluid also plays a role in removing waste from the brain and providing nutrients for its health. It flows through spaces within the brain and spinal cord called **ventricles**.

Think of CSF as a shield that keeps the brain and spinal cord healthy and functioning optimally. This is the same fluid that can be accessed through an epidural for the relief of pain associated with giving birth. CSF can also be collected during a spinal tap to assess for specific disorders such as meningitis.

This is where the BBB comes into play, as it regulates the passage of substances between the bloodstream and CSF and safeguards the brain by filtering out potentially harmful toxins or infectious organisms (bacteria or viruses) while permitting essential nutrients, including oxygen and glucose, to flow freely. One may wonder why we have a BBB in the first place rather than allowing the immune system free, unfettered access to the CNS. One reason is that the brain is susceptible to alterations in its surroundings. Think of neurons as divas that play a role in communication within the brain and require constant ions, nutrients, and signaling molecules for efficient operation.

Fluctuations in these levels can interfere with the brain's signals, resulting in issues such as seizures and damage to the brain.

Meanwhile, the primary role of the immune system is to directly target and eliminate threats such as bacteria or viruses. In a scenario where the immune system could freely penetrate the brain's boundaries, there is a risk that it could misidentify neurons, for example, as intruders and launch an attack against them by mistake.

Recall that the brain is unique compared to body tissues because it cannot regenerate or repair itself. Without the BBB, then, constant immune cell access could result in irreversible damage, leading to permanent loss of brain function. Therefore, the BBB is crucial to controlling the immune system's access to the brain.

What Comprises the BBB?

The BBB is a highly specialized structure composed of several key components that regulate what substances can pass from the blood into the brain. The two significant elements of the BBB are the **endothelial cells** and **astrocytes.**

Endothelial cells form the inner lining of capillaries in the CNS. Capillaries represent the smallest diameter vessels in the body, so small that red blood cells packed with oxygen must pass through in a single file. Every single one of your 35 trillion cells has access to a capillary. Capillaries are where nutrients and waste are exchanged through tiny slits or windows between the endothelial cells. These slit junctions are prominent in specific organs in the body, for example, the liver, the major metabolizing organ. Therefore, we say that capillaries that feed the liver are "leaky."

On the other hand, those slit junctions are *non-existent* in the CNS. There, the endothelial cells are packed together and form tight junctions, which create a near-impenetrable barrier. These tight junctions are composed of specialized proteins that seal endothelial cells tightly together, hence the name. This prevents more charged substances, toxins, and potentially harmful chemicals from passing out of the brain capillaries into the CSF, thus keeping the brain environment pristine.

The other major component, astrocytes, are numerous in the brain. Unlike neurons, astrocytes cannot generate electrical signals and have support roles in the CNS. One crucial function is helping form the BBB. The "end feet" of astrocytes wrap around blood vessels and contribute to the tightness of the barrier (Figure 9.1).

Collectively, tight junctions and astrocytes confer high selectivity, allowing certain substances, like nutrients (e.g., glucose, amino acids) and essential ions, to pass through the endothelial cells via specialized transport proteins while preventing, to a large extent, anything else. The BBB's tight junctions are like a VIP rope line at an exclusive club, with only the proper nutrients and small substances getting past the astrocytes playing bouncer. At the same time, the rest are left outside, wondering why they were not invited to the brain's inner party.

Figure 9.1: The Arrangement and Vital Elements of the BBB

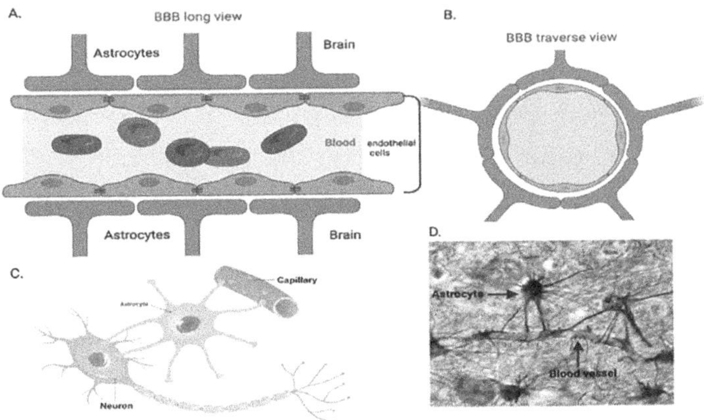

Note: The BBB safeguards the brain from substances in the bloodstream while permitting nutrients to enter smoothly. Panel A: A long view of the BBB showcases how blood circulates through the capillaries (blood vessels). The barrier is constructed by packed cells lining these capillaries' walls. Surrounding these capillaries are astrocyte cells (in purple), which uphold the integrity of the BBB and sustain brain function. Panel B illustrates a cross-sectional view of the blood-brain barrier, with a circular depiction of a blood vessel surrounded by astrocytes. Astrocytes extend their "feet" to enfold the vessels and provide support while regulating the flow of substances into the brain. Panel C depicts the connection between neurons (blue), astrocytes (yellow), and blood vessels, highlighting how astrocytes facilitate communication between capillaries and brain cells to maintain brain function. Panel D is an actual stained microscopic image in which dark-colored astrocytes envelop a blood vessel with their visible long extensions, interacting to uphold this protective barrier effectively and ensure the smooth passage of crucial nutrients and signals to the brain.

HOW CAN WE CIRCUMVENT THE BBB?

Although the BBB allows the brain to remain pristine and protected, it also poses a significant barrier to the development of CNS therapeutics, including CRISPR and RNA therapies. Whether administering a protein (e.g., Cas9), DNA, or RNA (e.g., gRNA or shRNA), these large, polar molecules cannot pass through the BBB. Therefore, any CNS therapeutic that is polar or large cannot be administered by the systemic intravenous route.

Injection and Its Drawbacks

What are the other alternatives? Options are limited and typically involve the injection of needles into the CNS. An intrathecal injection involves administering medication directly into the CSF that envelops the brain and spinal cord. This process involves inserting a long needle into the lower back region, known as the lumbar area, and explicitly targeting the *intrathecal space*, a fluid-filled region between the spinal cord and the nearby vertebrae.

Though intrathecal injections can serve as a method for delivering medication to the CNS, there are real risks linked to this process. Whenever a needle is inserted into the body, there is a chance of infection occurring, especially when it comes to injection, as bacteria or other harmful agents entering the CSF can result in infections such as meningitis. Another issue to be aware of is bleeding into the space or spinal cord that could cause compression of the cord and nerves, potentially resulting in serious complications. Additionally, following an injection procedure, some patients may develop a headache due to cerebrospinal fluid leakage at the puncture site, which can cause discomfort while standing but ease when lying down. These headaches can occasionally be very severe. Finally, although uncommon, there exists a possibility of nerve damage in case the needle comes into contact with or harms nerves in the region during the injection, leading to sensations of pain, numbness, or weakness.

For most people, the phrase "needle in the brain" lands somewhere between "hard pass" and "absolutely not"—even before they hear about the potential side effects. Administering medications to the brain and spinal cord through injections is a *relatively* good method that sidesteps the protective BBB limitations. However, if repeated doses are required, this is not an attractive route, and many patients may avoid therapy altogether due to the invasiveness of this procedure.

ANOTHER ALTERNATIVE: AAV9 VECTORS

To deliver our therapy to the brain and spinal cord, we use **AAV9 vectors**, which can be thought of as tiny FedEx trucks that deliver gene-editing tools to specific destinations. Of all the options available, AAV9 is considered one of the safest. It does not induce disease in humans and elicits mild immune responses (unlike other delivery trucks that might set off alarms in the body).

It also has a unique feature: it can penetrate the BBB. Although AAV9 works through this barrier slowly, it still does so effectively. A great example of AAV9 in action is Zolgensma, a gene therapy for **spinal muscular atrophy (SMA).** In the case of SMA, these delivery trucks release a functional *SMN1* gene to the motor neurons, the cells responsible for movement. This has been known to aid children with SMA by supporting better motor control and life expectancy.

Of course, every delivery system has its flaws. High doses of AAV9 may lead to hepatic toxicity, which is overloading the liver like a traffic jam at a busy hub. However, the advantages gained include better motor function and increased life expectancy. In addition, AAV9 trucks are very effective in reaching most parts of the brain and spinal cord; hence, they are suitable for targeting the neurons that require assistance (Meyer et al., 2015).

A BETTER SOLUTION

While traditional routes of administration, such as oral, intravenous, or intrathecal injections, present challenges in delivering therapeutics to the central nervous system, **intranasal delivery** offers a noninvasive and efficient alternative for bypassing the BBB. The development of noninvasive intranasal delivery platforms that effectively transport therapeutic compounds across the BBB, directly targeting neural circuits, has significantly enhanced the therapeutic efficacy of RNA therapeutics (Figure 9.2). This method represents a significant advancement over traditional gene-based interventions, which often require invasive intrathecal injections.

Figure 9.2: Nose-To-Brain Delivery of Gene Therapy Using AAV9 Vectors

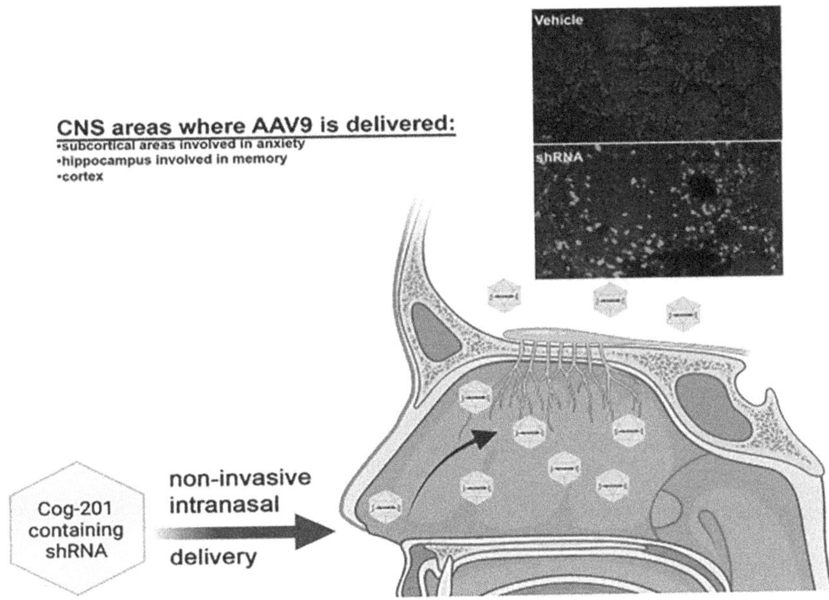

Note: The top right panel depicts the mouse brain image indicating delivery of Cog-201 into the brain as illustrated by the green labeling of neurons in the olfactory bulb. A color version of this figure can be found at getfitnow.com/extras.

Figure 9.2 illustrates the non-invasive delivery of a gene therapy (Cog-201) containing shRNA through the nasal passages into the brain. The treatment is administered intranasally, allowing the AAV9 (a type of viral vector) to travel directly to key brain areas, such as regions involved in anxiety, memory, and cognitive functions.

How can AAV9 cargo circumvent the BBB in this scenario? There are three major pathways by which material can enter the CNS following intranasal delivery (Hanson & Frey, 2008).

The first pathway involves **the olfactory bulb** (Figure 9.3). Medicinal substances or gene therapy carriers such as AAV9 can be transported into the brain via the nasal passage, utilizing the capabilities of the olfactory system. AAV9 vector particles interact with olfactory nerve cells in the nasal passage when delivered via intranasal delivery. These nerve cells are directly linked to the olfactory bulb at the base of the brain. This connection allows therapeutic substances to travel through the same pathways that process odors, reaching brain regions via these neural connections. This method allows treatments to be administered directly to brain areas, bypassing the BBB.

Figure 9.3: Nose-To-Brain Delivery of AAV9 Gene Therapy Via the Olfactory Pathway

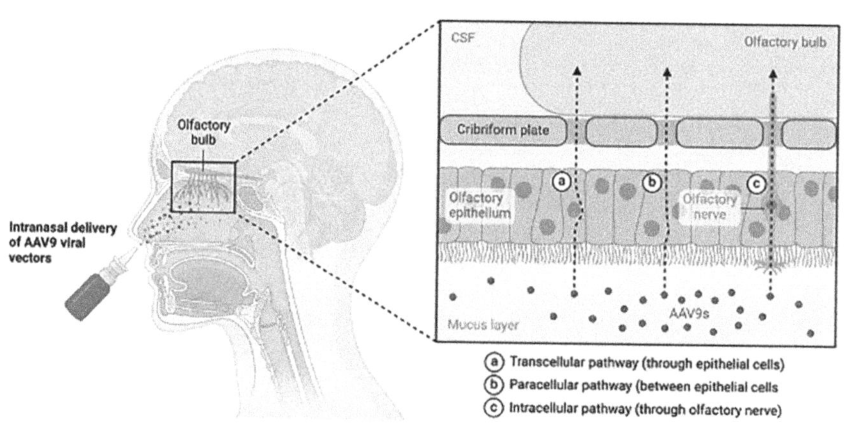

Figure 9.3 shows how AAV9 viral vectors, which carry shRNA, are delivered intranasally (through the nose) and can reach the brain. After being sprayed into the nose, the viral particles pass through the nasal cavity, where they come into contact with the olfactory epithelium, a tissue responsible for detecting smells. From here, the viral vectors can take different routes: they may pass directly through the cells, between the cells, or even travel along the olfactory nerve to reach the olfactory bulb, a brain region. This non-invasive delivery method targets the brain through natural pathways, providing a potential therapeutic approach for brain conditions.

The second pathway of entry involves the **trigeminal nerve**. The trigeminal nerve allows sensory information regarding the face and nose to travel to the brain for interpretation. The trigeminal nerve plays a role in causing those sudden headaches we get from eating ice cream too quickly, commonly known as “ice cream headaches.”

When something cold like ice cream comes into contact with the roof of the mouth or the back of the throat, it causes a rapid decrease in temperature in that spot. The brain perceives this as pain and wrongly associates it with the forehead or behind the eyes, resulting in the brief headache we call a “brain freeze.”

AAV9 viral particles infiltrate nerve endings and travel along these nerve fibers without crossing the blood-brain barrier (Figure 9.4). This alternative pathway from the trigeminal nerve allows cargo to reach deeper areas in the brainstem. The trigeminal nerve acts as a pathway from the nose to the brain, making it a crucial route for non-invasively delivering treatments to the brain.

Figure 9.4: Nose-To-Brain Biomolecule Delivery Via the Trigeminal Pathway

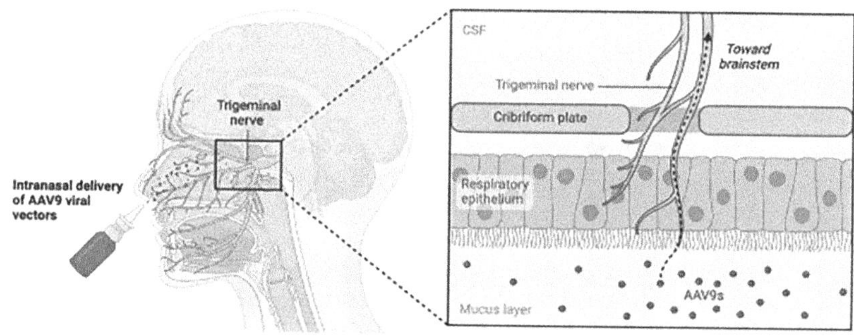

Note: This image shows how AAV9 viral vectors can be delivered to the brain through the trigeminal nerve pathway. Adapted from Jeong et al., 2023.

After the viral vectors are sprayed into the nose, they contact the mucous membrane in the nasal cavity. The trigeminal nerve, which senses sensations from the face and nasal area, has branches that extend into this region. The viral vectors can be taken up by the nerve endings and transported along the trigeminal nerve, eventually reaching deeper brain regions, including the brainstem. This non-invasive method allows the therapy to bypass the blood-brain barrier and target the brain through the trigeminal nerve's natural pathways.

Further delivery to the CNS occurs through the **rostral migratory stream (RMS).** Similar to how a conveyor belt efficiently moves products to their intended location swiftly and smoothly, the RMS navigates neuronal precursors straight to their required destination within the olfactory bulb.

Previous studies have demonstrated that intranasal administration of a fluorescent tracer allows agents to be distributed, in part via the RMS, throughout the entire brain, including the olfactory bulb, cortex, and cerebellum (Scranton et al., 2011).

ANTICIPATED BENEFITS

An intranasal platform like this offers a promising avenue for treating neurodegenerative and neuropsychiatric disorders (such as Alzheimer's disease or anxiety) with increased efficacy and safety over traditional delivery methods. Table 9.1 (continued on next page) compares gene therapy therapeutics such as CRISPR/Cas9, shRNA, and siRNA, considering the delivery routes and how they interact with the BBB.

Table 9.1: Comparison of Routes for Delivering Gene Therapy Therapeutics Beyond the Blood-Brain Barrier

GENE THERAPY	DELIVERY ROUTE	BBB PENETRATION	MECHANISM	ADVANTAGES	CHALLENGES
CRISPR/ Cas-9	Intrathecal (spinal injection)	High	Direct delivery into the cerebrospinal fluid (CSF) bypasses the BBB, allowing gene editing	Bypasses the BBB, precise gene editing in CNS cells (including neurons)	Invasive, requires surgical procedures, potential immune response, off-target effects
shRNA/ siRNA	Intranasal (nasal spray)	High (for certain drugs)	Bypasses the BBB through olfactory and trigeminal nerve pathways	Non-invasive, direct brain targeting, fewer systemic side effects	Limited drug types suitable for intranasal route, stability and formulation challenges, drug delivery efficiency

GENE THERAPY	DELIVERY ROUTE	BBB PENETRATION	MECHANISM	ADVANTAGES	CHALLENGES
shRNA/siRNA	Intravenous	Low	Drugs are injected directly into the bloodstream	Relatively non-invasive, safe, well-characterized route	Limited BBB penetration, requires delivery modifications (e.g. carriers), risk of systemic side effects

In summary, the intranasal delivery route offers the potential to deliver medications through the nasal passage, which allows access to the brain via the olfactory and trigeminal nerve pathways and the RMS without having to deal with crossing the BBB. Thus, the intranasal delivery of drugs offers a solution for enabling larger therapeutic molecules, such as RNA-based treatments or proteins, to reach the brain more efficiently, all without facing typical barriers.

There was a lot of detailed information in that last section! But I hope it helps you to understand the advantages of intranasal delivery and why evading the blood-brain barrier is important. By exploring intranasal delivery, we may one day develop anxiety treatments that go beyond the limitations of current small-molecule drugs, offering more direct and effective results with less adverse impact.

10

Navigating FDA Approval

Gene Therapy in Anxiety Treatment

HOW HAVE MEDICATIONS worked for me? My assessment is: "I have no idea."

I think it helps dampen the anxiety noise in my day-to-day life, but I do not believe it has much of an effect at all on acute anxiety situations. Doctors have offered hydroxyzine, an antihistamine and the only FDA-approved medication specifically for anxiety treatment. (It works by blocking histamine receptors in the brain.) While considered an excellent non-addictive alternative to benzodiazepines, one of the well-known side effects is marked drowsiness. The last thing I want to do at a Dave Matthews concert is take a nap!

This illustrates why I have dedicated myself to exploring new approaches to managing chronic anxiety: I believe there has to be a solution that targets both the persistent undercurrent nature of anxiety and those unexpected surges that disrupt daily routines. It is not just about enhancing my well-being but also about developing something that could support millions of individuals who are now struggling to balance the benefits of medication and its challenging side effects.

My personal experience with anxiety medications has been a frustrating exercise in compromise. The gap between what I require and what is available makes me more determined than ever to explore other alternatives that may be more suitable. However, even if we discover a new treatment, whether it is gene therapy or any other type of treatment, it is not all that easy to bring that treatment to patients.

In this chapter, I will explain the approval process that a novel therapy, such as gene therapy, must go through before being made available to patients. I'll discuss the scientific, regulatory, and financial aspects that must be considered and dealt with to ensure the therapy's safety and effectiveness. Understanding this journey is essential to appreciating how innovation becomes accessible to those who need it most.

Table 10.1 illustrates the time and cost of the entire approval process. Getting FDA approval is like convincing your cat to bathe—technically possible and legally necessary, but also a test of patience, fortitude, and luck.

Table 10.1: Evaluation Process for New Medical Treatments

STAGE	YEARS	MAJOR OBJECTIVE	POTENTIAL COST (USD)
Preclinical	6.5	Test drug safety and efficacy in animal models	$1–10 million
Phase I	1	Assess safety and dosage in a small group of healthy volunteers	$10–100 million
Phase II	2	Evaluate drug effectiveness and side effects in a larger group (100–200 subjects)	$100–200 million
Phase III	3	Confirm effectiveness, monitor side effects, and compare with standard treatments in a larger population (1,000–3,000 subjects)	$200–500 million
FDA	1–2	Review by FDA or equivalent regulatory agency for approval to market the drug	$2–5 million

OVERVIEW OF THE FDA

In the US, clinical trials are regulated by the Food and Drug Administration (FDA) to ensure that drugs reaching the market are both efficacious in treating the intended disorder or illness and safe for the intended patient population. Similar to many government regulatory agencies, the FDA evolved over time. In this regard, the FDA has weathered and been heavily influenced by catastrophic events ever since the passage of the Food and Drug Act in 1906. This Act dealt mainly with truth in labeling and empowered the FDA to remove any drug with an unknown composition. However, that act alone did not directly address drug safety or efficacy.

The tragic event known as the Elixir Sulfanilamide Disaster of 1937 was a watershed moment. During this incident, diethylene glycol (a component of antifreeze!) was "mistakenly" used as a solvent for sulfanilamide, an antibiotic then widely used. The pharmaceutical company behind this formulation believed that liquid medicine (with some raspberry flavoring) was more popular in the Southern U.S. However, they did *not* conduct safety tests on the final product due to a lack of requirements at that time. As a result of consuming this substance, more than 105 people, mostly children, lost their lives due to kidney failure (the oxalic acid introduced into their systems is highly toxic to the kidneys) (Marraffa et al., 2008).

The public uproar following this event was intense and led to the enactment of new laws, including the Food and Drug Administration Act of 1938. This Act ensured that drugs undergo safety testing before being approved for sale (Wax, 1995). It was this law that also spared the U.S. from the thalidomide tragedy that swept Europe in the 1960s.

However, despite these new regulatory guidelines, no laws were in place regarding drug efficacy, and extravagant claims were still being touted by pharmaceutical companies. To address this problem, in 1962, Congress gave the FDA the power to ensure drugs exhibited efficacy (or effectiveness) by passing the Kefauver-Harris Amendments. The Kefauver Harris Amendments required "evidence" (in other words, data, and not false claims) of effectiveness through conducted clinical trials. This change signified a noteworthy advancement in the FDA rules (Paine, 2017).

CLINICAL TRIALS

In the U.S., clinical trials are currently regulated by the FDA to ensure that drugs reaching the market are both efficacious in treating the intended disorder or illness and safe for the intended patient population (The FDA's Drug Review Process: Ensuring Drugs Are Safe and Effective, 2017). The odds are in favor of the agency, not the drug company.

The process for new drugs is divided into two sections: preclinical and clinical. The process typically spans 12-15 years, with costs ranging from $1 billion to over $2 billion per drug (DiMasi et al., 2016). Approximately five out of 5,000 new drugs complete the preclinical phase and advance to human clinical trials. Of those five, only one drug is typically approved by the FDA and reaches the marketplace (Dabrowska & Thaual, 2018).

After research and development, in the simplest case, the whole clinical trial process consists of distinct phases: preclinical, followed by Phases I-III of human clinical trials. Figure 10.1 depicts an overview of this entire process.

Figure 10.1: Drug Development in Four Phases

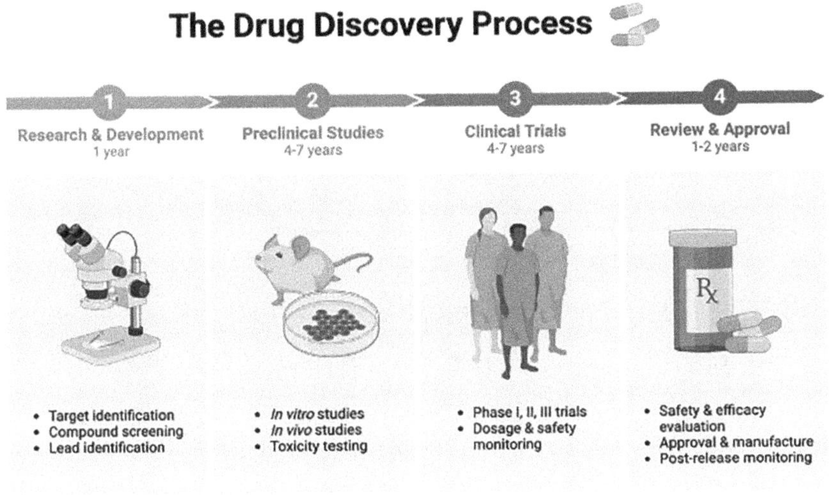

The Drug Discovery Process

1 Research & Development
1 year

2 Preclinical Studies
4-7 years

3 Clinical Trials
4-7 years

4 Review & Approval
1-2 years

- Target identification
- Compound screening
- Lead identification

- *In vitro* studies
- *In vivo* studies
- Toxicity testing

- Phase I, II, III trials
- Dosage & safety monitoring

- Safety & efficacy evaluation
- Approval & manufacture
- Post-release monitoring

Note: The four phases are research and development (R&D), preclinical studies, human clinical trials to assess the effectiveness and proper dosage levels, and review for official approval before being available to the public market.

THE PRE-CLINICAL PHASE

The process from synthesis of a new drug to its approval for use by patients may take 12–15 years, with the **preclinical phase** representing the longest running time, on average, at 6.5 years.

This phase has many components, including studies already discussed in this book, such as:

- In vitro models
- In vivo models examining target engagement
- Behavioral outcomes
- Proof-of-concept studies

At the preclinical stage, the risk-to-benefit ratio is determined by conducting **toxicity studies**. Additionally, the preclinical phase aims to gather information on the proposed drug's pharmacokinetics, chemistry, manufacturing plan, and potential quality control (Van Norman, 2016).

The finding of Viagra (also known as sildenafil) as a solution for erectile dysfunction stands out as a famous case where a medication was utilized for a different purpose. Designed for treating heart ailments, clinical studies unveiled another benefit: a significant improvement in the erectile function of male subjects participating in the trials was observed! In a surprise twist, this "little blue pill" would soon revolutionize sexual health and become a cultural phenomenon, forever changing the way we think about treatments and the power of scientific serendipity.

SUBMITTING THE APPLICATION: THE IND

The next step in the FDA drug-approval process is creating a **new investigational drug application (IND)** that, if approved, will permit sponsors to begin clinical trials. The IND application contains the necessary preclinical data for the FDA to assess and authorize testing in human subjects. This process allows the FDA to validate the medication's safety and effectiveness before clinical trials begin (Dreher-Lesnick et al., 2017).

After the IND is submitted, the FDA's Center for Drug Evaluation and Research (CDER) evaluates it. The CDER then assigns the application to the clinical review division according to the therapeutic area under study. This thorough review is meant to guarantee the scientific integrity of the proposed clinical trials while protecting the rights and well-being of those participating.

The duration of the IND process can differ based on the drug's complexity and the completeness of the application submitted for approval. Typically, the FDA allows 30 days to review and respond to IND submissions when they request more details or changes to the study plan (Van Norman, 2018). Following approval of the IND application, sponsors can commence trials.

Submitting an IND application is critical to bringing a drug to market. It allows new drugs to be tested in clinical trials while prioritizing participant safety. It is important to note that typically, a sponsor does not submit an IND application "cold turkey" to the FDA. Often, the sponsor will try to set up an INTERACT meeting. This meeting provides a chance for sponsors developing novel therapeutics to engage in consultations with the FDA. Sponsors usually request these meetings in the early stages of product development to receive advice regarding areas of their research program before submitting the IND application.

Meetings like these are crucial for cutting-edge or complex biological products, such as gene therapies and vaccines, because understanding the regulatory process early can significantly impact the success of the development plan. Unfortunately, the FDA denies around two-thirds of all INTERACT meeting requests, the most common reason being that the meeting request is submitted too early or too late in development. An INTERACT meeting with the FDA is like trying to schedule coffee with a celebrity. Most are either too early in their career for them to care or too late and already swamped with more exciting prospects.

FURTHER TESTING?

In some cases, it may be necessary to undergo further testing in non-human primates (NHPs), such as in old-world monkeys, before moving to human clinical trials. NHPs are often considered the most relevant animal models for evaluating the safety of new drugs due to their close genetic and physiological similarities to humans (Buckley et al., 2011).

This raises ethical issues surrounding NHPs' intelligence and their ability to display behaviors and feelings, a point frequently brought up in debates on animal experimentation. Numerous researchers and groups support practical methods for testing that do not involve using primates in biomedical research due to their cognitive and emotional capabilities.

In addition to ethical issues, there is also the issue of cost, which can quickly run into the millions of dollars for a single NHP study.

The FDA does not always mandate safety trials in NHPs for every new product under investigation; however, testing in NHPs may be suggested based on the type of therapeutic and study context involved, such as for biologics like gene therapies and vaccines. Why? Because NHPs closely mimic human physiology and immune responses, safety testing in primates may sometimes be necessary.

The FDA usually shows flexibility in its approach and advises sponsors to explain why they selected animal models using scientific reasoning. If there are scientific grounds for not using NHPs, alternative models may be considered, provided the sponsor can demonstrate that these alternatives can provide valuable safety information. The FDA assesses the sufficiency of safety data case by case.

One possible solution is the use of simulation software. For example, some companies offer bio-simulation services that use models to forecast how medications interact within the human body. Their methodology empowers pharmaceutical and biotech firms to make choices throughout the drug development journey.

Tools such as pharmacodynamic modeling systems, virtual populations, and regulatory science support can be modeled using computers to anticipate human responses to drugs, all using preclinical data, and can thereby sidestep the need for excessive animal experimentation. This modeling method can also generate simulated populations that replicate the range of body functions and characteristics, such as various demographics, genetics, and medical conditions.

Simulation software enables companies to evaluate safety and effectiveness through computer simulations rather than being compelled to conduct animal research, especially in NHPs. Additionally, these studies can be conducted at a fraction of the cost compared to NHP studies.

PHASE I OF HUMAN CLINICAL TRIALS

Following the approval of an IND by the FDA, clinical trials may begin in Phase I. Phase I clinical trials represent the first incidence of human exposure to the drug candidate. The sponsor typically focuses their efforts on testing in a small sample of healthy volunteers (<50), avoiding, for the time, adverse effects that may be unique to, or more extreme in, a diseased population (The FDA's Drug Review Process: Ensuring Drugs Are Safe and Effective, 2017).

Phase I studies are primarily safety trials to assess the toxicity and pharmacokinetic factors associated with the treatment (Williams, 2016). The primary objective is to assess the drug's safety by identifying any potential harmful side effects and establishing a safe dosage range for subsequent patient administration in testing phases.

Phase I also seeks to comprehend the drug's **pharmacokinetics** (that is, how the body processes a drug over time) and **pharmacodynamics** (in other words, how a drug interacts with its target in the body). Even though efficacy (also referred to as "effectiveness") is not the primary objective, the initial data on how the drug impacts functioning sometimes provides valuable insights for future developmental stages.

Although healthy volunteers are recruited for the majority of Phase I studies, in the case of life-threatening conditions like cancer, Phase I studies are frequently carried out directly involving individuals suffering from the ailment. This approach is taken because the treatment's effects and safety need to be assessed in the actual disease context. For this reason, there may be ethical concerns about exposing healthy people to potentially toxic drugs that are still under development.

PHASE II

Phase II trials are controlled clinical studies for 1) evaluating the drug's effectiveness in a specific disease and 2) defining an effective dose that provides the optimal benefit-risk profile for the use of the drug. Put differently, Phase II helps connect the dots between the theoretical understanding of the drug's action and its actual effect on behavior in the human brain.

In Phase II, studies are conducted on a larger scale (encompassing dozens to hundreds of patients) than in Phase I, working with patients who have the disorder the drug intends to treat. Phase II trials are typically divided into two parts: Phase IIa, which focuses on optimizing the dosage, and Phase IIb, which focuses on efficacy outcomes. Efficacy endpoints in Phase II trials can include clinical outcomes such as symptom improvement and surrogate endpoints (these are measurable changes believed to predict clinical benefit).

Safety assessment is a continual theme throughout the various phases of human clinical trials. Phase II includes side effects and more detailed pharmacokinetic and pharmacokinetic/dynamic information (that is, how the drug is metabolized and interacts with the body or brain). Based on these findings, an essential outcome of Phase II may be dose adjustments.

The average duration of this phase is two years, and after Phase II, the FDA and drug sponsors collaborate on Phase III study designs (Williams, 2016). It is noteworthy that 80 percent of all drugs tested are abandoned by their sponsors after Phase I or II because of excessive toxicity or lack of efficacy (Hollinger, 2007).

PHASE III

Phase III trials can be summarized as where "the rubber meets the road," as this is the last phase before FDA approval. Phase III studies are large, controlled clinical trials that involve thousands of people in the target disease population. The trials evaluate effectiveness, monitor side effects, and compare the drug with commonly used alternative therapies (Van Norman, 2016).

These studies also continue to assess the safety and efficacy of the proposed treatment; however, in Phase III, these assessments are conducted on a large enough scale to ensure that any observed results are statistically significant (Hollinger, 2007). A key aspect of phase III trials is that they must include enough patients to have at least an 80 percent chance of finding a clinical effect if it exists. This statistical feature of a clinical trial is often referred to as the **power of the study** (Hollinger, 2007).

An essential tenet of clinical trials, particularly in Phase III, is that they are **double-blind, placebo-controlled**. Double-blind refers to the concept that neither the researchers nor the patients know whether or not they are receiving the active ingredient.

These guardrails are in place to remove any potential bias. Guarding against the placebo effect is crucial, particularly when evaluating therapeutics that alter subjective experiences and behaviors within the brain.

A **placebo** is an inert treatment or substance without known effects in clinical studies. Researchers might utilize a placebo control group, and the impact of this placebo treatment is then compared to the results of the treated cohort. Even though placebos contain no active medication, researchers have found they can have a variety of both physical and psychological effects. Participants in placebo groups have displayed changes in, for example, heart rate, blood pressure, anxiety levels, pain perception, fatigue, and even brain activity.

One of the most studied and substantial placebo effects is in reducing pain. According to some estimates, approximately 30–60 percent of people will feel that their pain has diminished after taking a placebo pill. In this way, the placebo effect proves that sometimes our brains are just looking for an excuse to feel better; give them a "sugar pill," and they will throw a party like they have won the lottery.

FINAL STEP: THE NEW DRUG APPLICATION

Upon completing Phase III studies, researchers may submit a **New Drug Application (NDA)** to the FDA. This marks the beginning of an interim period, sometimes referred to as the FDA approval phase, which typically lasts one to two years. During this time, the FDA validates all previously collected data. The NDA formally requests the FDA to evaluate a drug's safety and approve it for sale in the U.S. (Williams, 2016). According to the Office of Federal Register 2024, the 2024 application fee for an NDA that requires clinical data was $4,048,695!

After an NDA is submitted, the FDA has 60 days to decide whether to accept it for review. In fact, the FDA reviews and acts on at least 90 percent of NDAs within ten months for standard drugs and within six months for priority drugs (Williams, 2016).

FUTURE APPLICATIONS OF GENE THERAPY

The age of personalized gene therapy is upon us. Its evolution from a science fiction plot to a tangible, real-world solution with the potential to revolutionize the treatment of anxiety and various neuropsychiatric conditions is genuinely remarkable.

However, as much as this book has been about the science behind gene therapies, it is also a deeply personal narrative about resilience, frustration, hope, and, ultimately, the belief that we are on the cusp of revolutionary change in medicine. Reflecting on the journey depicted in this book has made me realize how intricately connected my experiences and scientific endeavors have become. My struggles with anxiety and my relentless pursuit of novel treatment options have significantly fueled my dedication to this field of work.

The promise of gene therapy goes beyond treating symptoms; it delves into addressing the root causes of anxiety itself—a leap from merely managing the condition to potentially curing it altogether! Of course, with such breakthroughs come responsibilities. As we progress with these technological advancements, we must always be aware of ethical considerations and ensure that our actions protect safety and promote fairness for all individuals involved.

SUPPORTING RESEARCH AND DEVELOPMENT

Addressing health as a global concern is vital due to the widespread impact of anxiety disorders and the current limitations of conventional treatments. As we've seen, the costs of developing new therapies are substantial, and having sufficient financial resources is essential. Start-up gene therapy companies focused on mental health often attract philanthropic investors who aim to create meaningful and lasting change, as they see gene therapy as addressing a significant gap in available treatment options.

Regarding long-term goals and influence, these philanthropic capitalists tend to be more patient than conventional venture capitalists because they prioritize making a difference in society. For instance, they might be open to investing in RNA therapeutics at the early stages if they see their transformative potential for improving anxiety or memory impairments over time. Ultimately, donors with a penchant for innovation may be drawn to supporting groundbreaking technologies in this field, which promise to significantly enhance the quality of life for countless individuals.

Final Thoughts

I CONCLUDE THE BOOK *Brain Medicine* with great hope regarding the direction of mental health treatment. We have reached an exceptional inflexion in treating neuropsychiatric disorders, including anxiety, which enables us to both manage anxiety and possibly eliminate it through the combination of scientific progress, improved understanding, and compassionate care.

I have revealed my struggles with anxiety throughout this experience. My personal experiences with anxiety have driven me to discover new and effective treatment methods. The book presents the gene therapies that my team and I developed, known as Cog-101, alongside Cog-201. Cog-101 applies CRISPR to disable the *HTR2A* gene, which controls the expression of the 5-HT2A receptor responsible for anxiety, permanently. The approach of Cog-201 differs from Cog-101 because it utilizes RNA interference (RNAi) to reduce receptor production while maintaining DNA integrity. Our preclinical rodent research demonstrated that these treatments successfully diminished anxiety behaviors in laboratory settings. The Cog-201 therapy delivered a double advantage by both decreasing anxiety symptoms and enhancing memory performance. These results demonstrate the potential for a single-use gene therapy treatment of chronic anxiety that avoids the adverse effects of SSRIs.

The future path will present numerous obstacles to overcome. The process of obtaining FDA approval for gene therapy involves an extended sequence of expensive and complex steps. The path to gene therapy development faces substantial ethical dilemmas regarding how to distribute access to patients while maintaining safety standards. Our progress requires us to balance scientific progress with moral decisions that protect public trust. The future of gene therapy for mental health will advance through scientific progress, policymakers' action, ethical considerations, and societal acceptance of new possibilities.

The current obstacles require effort to defeat, but scientists now possess tools to treat mental health disorders through genetic intervention. Modern genetic tools enable medical professionals to identify and treat biological factors that cause anxiety and depression and their associated mental health conditions. The new therapeutic approaches function as additional treatment options because counseling, medication, mindfulness, and supportive relationships continue to play a vital role in mental health care. The therapeutic field advances through new interventions that demonstrate potential to deliver enduring benefits to patients who fail to find relief from current treatments. The future of mental health treatment will evolve from symptom management to complete prevention and cure through the integration of advanced techniques with empathetic patient care.

The development of brain medicine combines scientific discoveries with human experiences. My personal experience with anxiety and my scientific research for solutions have shown that human progress emerges from the combination of being open and never giving up. The process of sharing my personal experiences has proven equally crucial to sharing research data because both demonstrate the need for improved mental health treatments. The future of mental health development depends on both technological progress and human empathy and personal strength that people show toward each other.

For additional content and full color illustrations, visit Brain Medicine at https://getfitnow.com/extras/

Glossary

5-HT2A receptor: a specific receptor for serotonin, which is a neurotransmitter implicated in anxiety, depression, memory, and other neuropsychiatric disorders.

AAV9 Vectors: a type of viral vector used to deliver genetic material into cells, commonly employed in gene therapy.

ADHD (Attention Deficit Hyperactivity Disorder): a neurodevelopmental disorder characterized by patterns of inattention, hyperactivity, and impulsivity that interfere with functioning or development.

Amygdala: a part of the brain involved in emotion processing, particularly fear and anxiety.

Anxiety Disorder: a group of mental health conditions characterized by excessive fear, worry, and behavioral disturbances.

AON (Antisense Oligonucleotide): short, synthetic strands of DNA or RNA designed to bind to specific mRNA molecules to alter gene expression, often used in gene silencing therapies.

AUG (Start Codon): a specific sequence of RNA that signals the beginning of protein synthesis, coding for the amino acid methionine.

Blood-Brain Barrier (BBB): a selective barrier that protects the brain from harmful substances while allowing essential nutrients to pass through.

Cas9: a protein associated with the CRISPR system, functioning as molecular scissors to cut DNA at specific locations.

Central Dogma of Molecular Biology: the process of genetic information flowing from DNA to RNA to protein.

Codons: triplets of nucleotides in mRNA that specify particular amino acids or signal the start or stop of protein synthesis.

CRISPR (Clustered Regularly Interspaced Short Palindromic Repeats): a revolutionary gene-editing tool that allows scientists to make precise changes to DNA, often paired with the Cas9 protein.

Diazepam: a medication used to treat anxiety, muscle spasms, and seizures, often sold under the brand name Valium.

DNA (Deoxyribonucleic Acid): the molecule that carries genetic information in all living organisms, composed of two strands forming a double helix.

Downregulation: a process by which a cell decreases the quantity of a specific molecule, such as a receptor or protein.

DSM-V: the *Diagnostic and Statistical Manual of Mental Disorders* (5th edition), used by clinicians for diagnosing mental health conditions.

Exon: a segment of a gene that codes for a portion of a protein.

Frameshift Disorder: a genetic condition caused by insertions or deletions in DNA that alter the reading frame of a gene.

GABA (Gamma-Aminobutyric Acid): an inhibitory neurotransmitter that reduces neuronal excitability, helping to calm the brain and alleviate anxiety.

Gene Expression: the process by which genetic information is used to produce proteins essential for cell function and response to the environment.

Gene Silencing: the process of reducing or completely shutting down the expression of a specific gene, preventing it from producing its corresponding protein. This can be achieved through CRISPR, which introduces targeted changes to the DNA sequence to permanently disrupt the gene, or RNA interference (RNAi), which temporarily blocks the gene's messenger RNA (mRNA) to suppress protein production without altering the DNA.

Gene Therapy: a medical technique that uses genetic material to treat or prevent disease by inserting, altering, or silencing genes within an individual's cells.

Genes: segments of DNA that encode instructions for producing proteins or regulating biological processes.

Guide RNA: a short RNA sequence used in CRISPR to direct the Cas9 protein to specific DNA sites for editing.

Half-life: the time it takes for half of a substance (like a protein or drug) to degrade or be eliminated from the body.

Homology-directed repair (HDR): a precise DNA repair process using a template to fix double-stranded breaks.

Hydrophilic: describes molecules or substances that interact well with water.

Hyperactive Distressive Connectome: a posited network of neural pathways controlling the storage of dysfunctional memories, the processing of negative experiences, and the generation of maladaptive responses

In vitro: experiments conducted outside a living organism, typically in a controlled laboratory environment.

In vivo: experiments conducted within a living organism.

Intron: a non-coding segment of a gene that is removed during RNA splicing.

Investigational Drug Application (IND): a request submitted to regulatory agencies to begin clinical trials of a new drug.

mRNA (Messenger RNA): a type of RNA that carries genetic instructions from DNA to ribosomes for protein synthesis.

Mutation: a change in the DNA sequence that can affect gene function or expression.

Neuronal Spiking Activity: electrical signals generated by neurons to communicate with each other and process information.

Neurons: specialized cells in the nervous system that transmit information through electrical and chemical signals.

New Drug Application (NDA): a formal proposal for regulatory approval to market a new pharmaceutical in a country.

Non-Homologous End Joining (NHEJ): a quicker but

error-prone DNA repair mechanism that directly joins broken DNA ends.

Neurotransmitter: chemical messengers that transmit signals across synapses between neurons, influencing mood, behavior, and other physiological processes.

Prefrontal Cortex: the brain region associated with complex behaviors, decision-making, and emotional regulation.

Receptor: a protein molecule on a cell's surface or inside that binds to specific substances (neurotransmitters) to trigger a cellular response.

Reading Frame: how nucleotides in DNA or RNA are grouped into codons for translation into proteins.

Ribosomes: cellular structures located in the cytoplasm (hardhat zone) of cells where proteins are synthesized from mRNA instructions.

RNA (Ribonucleic Acid): a molecule essential for various biological roles, including coding, decoding, regulation, and expression of genes.

RNA Interference (RNAi): a biological process where RNA molecules inhibit gene expression by destroying specific mRNA molecules.

Serotonin: a neurotransmitter involved in mood regulation, anxiety, and other physiological functions.

shRNA (Short Hairpin RNA): a synthetic RNA molecule that silences specific genes by interfering with their mRNA.

siRNA (Small Interfering RNA): short, double-stranded RNA molecules that degrade mRNA to reduce or inhibit gene expression.

SSRIs (Selective Serotonin Reuptake Inhibitors): a class of medications that increase serotonin levels in the brain, commonly used to treat depression and anxiety.

References

Chapter 1

Baldwin, D. S., Aitchison, K., Bateson, A., Curran, H. V., Davies, S., Leonard, B., Nutt, D. J., Stephens, D. N., & Wilson, S. (2013). Benzodiazepines: risks and benefits. A reconsideration. *J Psychopharmacol, 27*(11), 967-971. https://doi.org/10.1177/0269881113503509

Cai, C., Woolhandler, S., Himmelstein, D. U., & Gaffney, A. (2021). Trends in anxiety and depression symptoms during the COVID-19 pandemic: Results from the

U.S. Census Bureau's Household Pulse Survey. *Journal of General Internal Medicine, 36*(6), 1841-1843. https://doi.org/10.1007/s11606-021-06759-9

Jakubovski, E., Johnson, J. A., Nasir, M., Muller-Vahl, K., & Bloch, M. H. (2019). Systematic review and meta-analysis: Dose-response curve of SSRIs and SNRIs in anxiety disorders. *Depress Anxiety, 36*(3), 198-212. https://doi.org/10.1002/da.22854

Lass-Hennemann, J., Peyk, P., Streb, M., Holz, E., & Michael, T. (2014). The presence of a dog reduces subjective but not physiological stress responses to an analog trauma. *Frontiers in Psychology, 5,* 1010. https://doi.org/10.3389/fpsyg.2014.01010

Leighton, S. C., Rodriguez, K. E., Jensen, C. L., MacLean, E. L., Davis, L. W., Ashbeck, E. L.,…O'Haire, M. E. (2024). Service dogs for veterans and military members with posttraumatic stress disorder: a nonrandomized controlled trial. *JAMA Network Open*, *7*(6), e2414686. https://doi.org/10.1001/jamanetworkopen.2024.14686

Olfson, M., King, M., & Schoenbaum, M. (2015). Benzodiazepine use in the United States. *JAMA Psychiatry*, *72*(2), 136-142. https://doi.org/10.1001/jamapsychiatry.2014.1763

Strawn, J. R., Welge, J. A., Wehry, A. M., Keeshin, B., & Rynn, M. A. (2015). Efficacy and tolerability of antidepressants in pediatric anxiety disorders: a systematic review and meta-analysis. *Depress Anxiety*, *32*(3), 149-157. https://doi.org/10.1002/da.22329

Suresh, V., Mills, J. A., Croarkin, P. E., & Strawn, J. R. (2020). What next? A Bayesian hierarchical modeling re-examination of treatments for adolescents with selective serotonin reuptake inhibitor-resistant depression. *Depress Anxiety*, *37*(9), 926-934. https://doi.org/10.1002/da.23064

Twenge, J. M., McAllister, C., & Joiner, T. E. (2021). Anxiety and depressive symptoms in U.S. Census Bureau assessments of adults: Trends from 2019 to fall 2020 across demographic groups. *Journal of Anxiety Disorders*, *83*, 102455. https://doi.org/10.1016/j.janxdis.2021.102455

Yarborough, B. J. H., Stumbo, S. P., Yarborough, M. T., Owen-Smith, A., & Green, C. A. (2018). Benefits and challenges of using service dogs for veterans with posttraumatic stress disorder. *Psychiatric Rehabilitation Journal*, *41*(2), 118-124. https://doi.org/10.1037/prj0000294

Chapter 2

Berger, M., Gray, J. A., & Roth, B. L. (2009). The expanded biology of serotonin. *Annual Review of Medicine*, *60*, 355-366. https://doi.org/10.1146/annurev.med.60.042307.11080 2

Cohen, H. (2005). Anxiolytic effect and memory improvement in rats by antisense oligodeoxynucleotide to 5-hydroxytryptamine-2A precursor protein. *Depression and Anxiety*, *22*(2), 84–93. https://doi.org/10.1002/da.20087

Erberk-Ozen, N. (2008). Manic symptoms are probably associated with short-term low-dose quetiapine use. *Advances in Therapy*, *25*(1), 53-58. https://doi.org/10.1007/s12325-008-0003-4

Fluyau, D., Revadigar, N., & Manobianco, B. E. (2018). Challenges of the pharmacological management of benzodiazepine withdrawal, dependence, and discontinuation. *Ther Adv Psychopharmacol*, *8*(5), 147-168. https://doi.org/10.1177/2045125317753340

Mackinnon, J.B. (2016, August 3). *The strange brain of the world's greatest solo climber.* Nautilus. https://nautil.us/the-strange-brain-of-the-worlds-greatest-solo-climber-236051/.

Weisstaub, N. V., Zhou, M., Lira, A., Lambe, E., Gonzalez-Maeso, J., Hornung, J. P. Gingrich, J. A. (2006). Cortical 5-HT2A receptor signaling modulates anxiety-like behaviors in mice. *Science*, *313*(5786), 536–540. https://doi.org/10.1126/science.1123432

Xiang, M., Jiang, Y., Hu, Z., Yang, Y., Botchway, B. O. A., & Fang, M. (2017). Stimulation of anxiety-like behavior via ERK pathway by competitive serotonin receptors 2A and 1A in post-traumatic stress disordered mice. *Neurosignals*, *25*(1), 39-53. https://doi.org/10.1159/000481791

Chapter 3

Unschuld, P. G., Ising, M., Erhardt, A., Lucae, S., Kloiber, S., Kohli, M., Salyakina, D., Welt, T., Kern, N., Lieb, R., Uhr, M., Binder, E. B., Muller-Myhsok, B., Holsboer, F., & Keck, M. E. (2007). Polymorphisms in the serotonin receptor gene HTR2A are associated with quantitative traits in panic disorder. *Am J Med Genet B Neuropsychiatry Genet*, *144B*(4), 424-429. https://doi.org/10.1002/ajmg.b.30412

Vermeire, S. T., Audenaert, K. R., Dobbeleir, A. A., De Meester, R. H., De Vos, F. J., & Peremans, K. Y. (2009). Evaluation of the brain 5-HT2A receptor binding index in dogs with anxiety disorders, measured with 123I-5I-R91150 and SPECT. *J Nucl Med*, *50*(2), 284-289. https://doi.org/10.2967/jnumed.108.055731

Chapter 4

Tanabe, P., Spratling, R., Smith, D., Grissom, P., & Hulihan, M. (2019). CE: Understanding the Complications of Sickle Cell Disease. *Am J Nurs*, *119*(6), 26-35. https://doi.org/10.1097/01.NAJ.0000559779.40570.2c

US Food and Drug Administration (FDA). (2023, December 8). *FDA approves first gene therapies to treat patients with sickle cell disease.* Author. https://www.fda.gov/news-events/press-announcements/fda-approves-first-gene-therapies-treat-patients-sickle-cell-disease#:~:text=Casgevy%2C%20a%20cell%2Dbased%20gene,DNA%20where%20it%20was%20cut.

Chapter 5

Dragt, Esmée, & Ngai, Louis (2017).Using CRISPR in your experiments. In *CRISPR 101: A Desktop Resource* (pp. 30-93). Addgene.

Jinek, M., Chylinski, K., Fonfara, I., Hauer, M., Doudna, J. A., & Charpentier, E. (2012). A programmable dual-RNA-guided DNA endonuclease in adaptive bacterial immunity. *Science, 337*(6096), 816-821. https://doi.org/10.1126/science.1225829

Rohn, T. T., Kim, N., Isho, N. F., & Mack, J. M. (2018). The Potential of CRISPR/Cas9 Gene Editing as a Treatment Strategy for Alzheimer's Disease. *J Alzheimers Dis Parkinsonism*, *8*(3). https://doi.org/10.4172/2161-0460.1000439

Yang, S., Chang, R., Yang, H., Zhao, T., Hong, Y., Kong, H. E.,… Li, X. J. (2017). CRISPR/Cas9-mediated gene editing ameliorates neurotoxicity in mouse models of Huntington's disease. *Journal of Clinical Investigation*, *127*(7), 2719–2724. https://doi.org/10.1172/JCI92087

Chapter 6

Fattouh, N., Hallit, S., Salameh, P., Choueiry, G., Kazour, F., & Hallit, R. (2019). Prevalence and factors affecting the level of depression, anxiety, and stress in hospitalized patients with a chronic disease. Perspectives in Psychiatric Care, 55(4), 592-599. https://doi.org/10.1111/ppc.12369

Kim, J. S., Park, J., Choi, J. H., Kang, S., & Park, N. (2023). RNA-DNA hybrid nano-materials for highly efficient and long-lasting RNA interference effect. RSC Adv*ances,* 13(5), 3139-3146. https://doi.org/10.1039/d2ra06249f

Pasi, K. J., Rangarajan, S., Georgiev, P., Mant, T., Creagh, M. D., Lissitchkov, T., Ragni, M. V. (2017). Targeting of antithrombin in hemophilia A or B with RNAI therapy. *New England Journal of Medicine, 377*(9), 819-828. https://doi.org/10.1056/NEJMoa1616569

Chapter 7

Rohn, T. T., Radin, D., Brandmeyer, T., Linder, B. J., Andriambeloson, E., Wagner, S., Kehler, J., Vasileva, A., Wang, H., Mee, J. L., & Fallon, J. H. (2023). Genetic modulation of the HTR2A gene reduces anxiety-related behavior in mice. *PNAS Nexus, 2*(6), pgad170. https://doi.org/10.1093/pnasnexus/pgad170

Santomauro, D. F., Herrera, A. M. M., Shadid, J., Zheng, P., Ashbaugh, C., Pigott, D. M. et al. (2021). "Global prevalence and burden of depressive and anxiety disorders in 204 countries and territories in 2020 due to the COVID-19 pandemic." *The Lancet, 378,* no. 10312, 1700-1712.

Chapter 8

Cohen, H. (2005). Anxiolytic effect and memory improvement in rats by antisense oligodeoxynucleotide to 5-hydroxytryptamine-2A precursor protein. *Depression and Anxiety, 22*(2), 84–93. https://doi.org/10.1002/da.20087

Poyurovsky, M., Koren, D., Gonopolsky, I., Schneidman, M., Fuchs, C., Weizman, A., & Weizman, R. (2003). Effect of the 5-HT2 antagonist mianserin on cognitive dysfunction in chronic schizophrenia patients: an add-on, double-blind placebo-controlled study. *European Neuropsychopharmacology, 13*(2), 123-128. https://doi.org/10.1016/s0924-977x(02)00155-4

Rohn, T. T., Radin, D., Brandmeyer, T., Seidler, P. G., Linder, B. J., Lytle, T., Macciardi, F. (2024a). Intranasal delivery of shRNA to knock down the 5HT-2A receptor enhances memory and alleviates anxiety. *Translational Psychiatry, 14*(1), 154. https://doi.org/10.1038/s41398-024-02879-y

Rohn, T. T., Radin, D., Brandmeyer, T., Seidler, P. G., Linder, B. J., Lytle, T., Macciardi, F. (2024b). Treatment with shRNA to knock down the 5-HT2A receptor improves memory in vivo and decreases excitability in primary cortical neurons. *Genomic Psychiatry.* https://doi.org/https://doi.org/10.61373/gp024r.0043

Zhang, G., & Stackman, R. W., Jr. (2015). The role of serotonin 5-HT2A receptors in memory and cognition. *Frontiers in Pharmacology, 6*, 225. https://doi.org/10.3389/fphar.2015.00225

Chapter 9

Hanson, L. R., & Frey, W. H., 2nd. (2008). Intranasal delivery bypasses the blood-brain barrier to target therapeutic agents to the central nervous system and treat neurodegenerative disease. *BMC Neuroscience, 9 Suppl 3*, S5. https://doi.org/10.1186/1471-2202-9-S3-S5

Jeong, S. H., Jang, J. H., & Lee, Y. B. (2023). Drug delivery to the brain via the nasal route of administration: exploration of key targets and major consideration factors. *Journal of Pharmaceutical Investigation*, *53*(1), 119-152. https://doi.org/10.1007/s40005-022-00589-5

Meyer, K., Ferraiuolo, L., Schmelzer, L., Braun, L., McGovern, V., Likhite, S.,...Kaspar, B. K. (2015). Improving single injection CSF delivery of AAV9-mediated gene therapy for SMA: a dose-response study in mice and nonhuman primates. *Molecular Therapy*, *23*(3), 477-487. https://doi.org/10.1038/mt.2014.210

Pardridge, W. M. (2005). The blood-brain barrier: bottleneck in brain drug development. *NeuroRx*, *2*(1), 3–14. https://doi.org/10.1602/neurorx.2.1.3

Scranton, R. A., Fletcher, L., Sprague, S., Jimenez, D. F., & Digicaylioglu, M. (2011). The rostral migratory stream plays a key role in the intranasal delivery of drugs into the CNS. *PLoS One*, *6*(4), e18711. https://doi.org/10.1371/journal.pone.0018711

Chapter 10

Buckley, L. A., Chapman, K., Burns-Naas, L. A., Todd, M. D., Martin, P. L., & Lansita, J. A. (2011). Considerations regarding nonhuman primate use in safety assessment of biopharmaceuticals. *International Journal of Toxicology, 30*(5), 583–590. https://doi.org/10.1177/1091581811415875

Dabrowska, A., & Thaual, S. (2018). *How the FDA approves drugs and regulates their safety and effectiveness.* US Food and Drug Administration. *http://www. fda.gov/Drugs/ResourcesForYou/Consumers/ucm1435 34.htm.*

DiMasi, J. A., Grabowski, H. G., & Hansen, R. W. (2016). Innovation in the pharmaceutical industry: new estimates of R&D costs. *Journal of Health Economics, 47*, 20-33. https://doi.org/10.1016/j.jhealeco.2016.01.012

Dreher-Lesnick, S. M., Stibitz, S., & Carlson, P. E., Jr. (2017). U.S. regulatory considerations for development of live biotherapeutic products as drugs. *Microbiology Spectrum, 5*(5). https://doi.org/10.1128/microbiolspec.BAD-0017-2017

Hollinger, M. A. (2007). Pharmaceutical development of drugs and the FDA. In *Introduction to Pharmacology* (3rd ed., pp. 317-331). CRC Press, Taylor & Francis Group.

Marraffa, J. M., Holland, M. G., Stork, C. M., Hoy, C. D., & Hodgman, M. J. (2008). Diethylene glycol: a widely used solvent that presents serious poisoning potential. *J Emerg Med, 35*(4), 401–406. https://doi.org/10.1016/j.jemermed.2007.06.025

Paine, M. F. (2017). Therapeutic disasters that hastened safety testing of new drugs. *Clin Pharmacol Ther, 101*(4), 430-434. https://doi.org/10.1002/cpt.613 *The FDA's Drug Review Process: Ensuring Drugs Are Safe and Effective.* (2017). U.S. Food and Drug Administration.

Van Norman, G. A. (2016). Drugs, devices, and the FDA: part 1: an overview of approval processes for drugs. *JACC: Basic to Translational Science, 1*(3), 170-179. https://doi.org/10.1016/j.jacbts.2016.03.002

Van Norman, G. A. (2018). Expanding patient access to investigational new drugs: overview of intermediate and widespread treatment investigational new drugs, and emergency authorization in public health emergencies. *JACC: Basic to Translational Science, 3*(3), 403-414. https://doi.org/10.1016/j.jacbts.2018.02.001

Wax, P. M. (1995). Elixirs, diluents, and the passage of the 1938 Federal Food, Drug, and Cosmetic Act. *Annals of Internal Medicine, 122*(6), 456–461. https://doi.org/10.7326/0003-4819-122-6-199503150-00009

Williams, C. T. (2016). Food and Drug Administration drug approval process: a history and overview. *Nursing Clinics of North America, 51*(1), 1–11. https://doi.org/10.1016/j.cnur.2015.10.007

Acknowledgments

THIS BOOK WOULD not have been possible without the incredible team I have had the pleasure to work with these past five-plus years.

My deepest thanks go to our Cognigenics team: Dean Radin, Tracy Brandmeyer, Peter Seidler, David Hitt, Tom Lytle, and Fabio Macciardi for their input and expertise in all matters related to the science of this book.

I am immensely grateful to John L. Mee and Barry Linder for allowing me to develop our preclinical program. My profound respect and admiration go to James Fallon, who taught me so much.

Finally, to my wife, Lisa, for her steadfast support, and to my children for putting up with a quirky, nerdy, and sometimes neurotic dad, I give my heartfelt love.

About the Author

Troy Rohn, PhD, has built a substantial academic reputation with nearly three decades of experience in neuroscience research and teaching. For his contributions to Alzheimer's research and neurological disorders, he was recently recognized as one of the top 0.5% of scholars worldwide. Dr. Rohn received his Ph.D. in Pharmacology from the University of Washington, Seattle. He had several Postdoctoral stints including two-plus years living in Paris, France, one year at Montana State University in Bozeman, Montana, and two years at UC Irvine. He has obtained extramural funding continuously since his arrival at Boise State University (where he currently works as a professor in the Biology Department) including grants from NIH, AFAR, and AHAF. Dr. Rohn has authored over 80 peer-reviewed publications, many of which address topics related to neurobiology, mental health, and treatment strategies.

NOTES